DUMMIES TYPE 2 DIABETES

A Comprehensive Guide to Understanding, Managing, and Living Well with Diabetes

JESSICA B TONY

TABLE OF CONTENT

Introduction   9
  Understanding Type 2 Diabetes: A Key to
  Empowerment   11
  - How to Use This Book   14
Chapter 1:   16
  1.1 What is Type 2 Diabetes?   16
  1.2 Causes and Risk Factors of Type 2 Diabetes 25
  1.3 Recognizing the Symptoms   36
  1.4 Getting Diagnosed   45
Chapter 2:   57
  - Managing Your Diabetes   57
  2.1 Monitoring Blood Sugar Levels   60
  2.2 Medication and Insulin Therapy   69
  2.3 Diet and Nutrition   82
  2.4 Exercise and Physical Activity   96
Chapter 3:   112
  Living Well with Diabetes   112
  3.1 Creating a Diabetes Management Plan   116
  3.2 Coping with the Emotional Impact   128
  3.3 Preventing Complications   141
  3.4 Navigating Social Situations   154
Chapter 4:   166
  4.1 Understanding the Latest Research   166
  4.2 Technological Tools for Diabetes Management182
  4.3 Personalized Medicine   197

Introduction

Welcome to *Type 2 Diabetes For Dummies*! Whether you've been recently diagnosed, have been managing diabetes for years, or are supporting a loved one, this book is here to guide you through the complexities of Type 2 diabetes with clarity and practical advice.

Type 2 diabetes is a chronic condition that affects the way your body metabolizes sugar (glucose), an essential energy source. Unlike Type 1 diabetes, where the body does not produce insulin, Type 2 diabetes is characterized by insulin resistance, meaning your body doesn't use insulin efficiently. Over time, your body may also produce less insulin. This can lead to elevated blood sugar levels, which, if unmanaged, can cause serious health complications.

To effectively manage Type 2 diabetes, one must first grasp the condition. This book breaks down medical jargon into plain English, providing you with the knowledge and tools needed to take control of your health. We'll explore what causes Type 2 diabetes, how it's diagnosed, and the common symptoms to watch for. But knowing about diabetes is only part of the journey. Managing it requires a holistic approach. You'll learn how to monitor your blood sugar, the role of medication and insulin, and the importance of diet and exercise. Additionally, this book covers the emotional and psychological aspects of living with diabetes, offering tips on stress management and finding support. We'll also delve into advanced topics, including the latest research, technological tools for diabetes management, and personalized treatment options. Whether you're newly diagnosed or looking for ways to optimize your current management plan, *Type 2 Diabetes For Dummies* is your go-to resource for living well with diabetes. Let's embark on this journey together, empowering you to lead a healthier, more informed life.

Understanding Type 2 Diabetes: A Key to Empowerment

Type 2 diabetes is a complex and multifaceted condition that affects millions worldwide. At its core, it is a metabolic disorder characterized by insulin resistance, impaired glucose regulation, and a range of associated complications. However, it is more than just a medical diagnosis – it is a call to action, an opportunity to take control of one's health and wellbeing.

To truly understand type 2 diabetes is to grasp the intricate interplay between lifestyle, genetics, and environment. It is to recognize the critical role that diet, physical activity, and stress management play in regulating blood sugar levels and mitigating the risk of long-term complications. It is to acknowledge the emotional and psychological toll of living with a chronic condition, and to seek support and resources when needed.

Perhaps most importantly, understanding type 2 diabetes is to empower oneself with knowledge, resilience, and hope. It is to recognize that small changes can add up to make a big difference, that every healthy choice is a step in the right direction, and that a diagnosis is not a definition. By embracing this understanding, individuals can break free from the grip of type 2 diabetes and reclaim navigate your new reality. You'll learn about the basics of the disease, the importance of blood sugar monitoring, and how to make lifestyle changes that can improve your health and quality of life.

For Those Managing Diabetes Long-Term
If you've been managing Type 2 diabetes for some time, this book offers advanced strategies to

- Who This Book is For
Type 2 Diabetes For Dummies is designed for anyone looking to understand and manage Type 2 optimize your care. From the latest research and technological tools to personalized treatment options, you'll find information that can help you refine your management plan and stay motivated on your journey to better health.

For Family Members and Caregivers

Supporting someone with Type 2 diabetes requires understanding the condition and its challenges. This book provides caregivers and family members with practical advice on how to offer support, recognize signs of complications, and assist in managing daily routines. By understanding what your loved one is going through, you can better help them lead a healthier, more fulfilling life.

For Health Enthusiasts and Educators

Health professionals, educators, and anyone interested in learning more about Type 2 diabetes will find this book to be a comprehensive guide. It covers the latest advancements in diabetes care, dietary guidelines, and exercise recommendations, making it a useful tool for teaching others about the condition.

For Those Seeking Prevention Strategies

Even if you don't have Type 2 diabetes but are at risk or simply want to prevent it, this book is for you. It outlines risk factors, preventive measures, and lifestyle changes that can significantly reduce your chances of developing the disease.

No matter your relationship to Type 2 diabetes, this book aims to empower you with knowledge, practical tips, and a supportive approach to managing and understanding the condition. Together, let's go out on this path to a better, more knowledgeable living.

- How to Use This Book

Type 2 Diabetes For Dummies is structured to provide you with a comprehensive, easy-to-navigate guide to understanding and managing Type 2 diabetes. Here's how to make the most out of this book:

Start with the Basics

If you're new to Type 2 diabetes, begin with Chapter 1: "The Basics of Type 2 Diabetes." This section covers the essential information about the condition, including what it is, its causes, symptoms, and how it's diagnosed. Knowing the basics will provide you with a strong base on which to develop.

Focus on Management

Once you're familiar with the basics, move on to Chapter 2: "Managing Your Diabetes." This chapter is packed with practical advice on monitoring blood sugar levels, medications, insulin therapy, diet, nutrition, and exercise. You'll find step-by-step guides and tips to help you integrate these management strategies into your daily routine.

Enhance Your Lifestyle

Chapter 1:

1.1 What is Type 2 Diabetes?

Chronic metabolic disease known as type 2 diabetes is typified by elevated blood sugar levels, resistance to insulin, and a relative lack of insulin. Unlike Type 1 diabetes, where the body's immune system attacks and destroys insulin-producing cells in the pancreas, Type 2 diabetes develops primarily due to a combination of genetic predisposition and lifestyle factors.

In Type 2 diabetes, the body becomes resistant to the effects of insulin, a hormone produced by the pancreas. Because insulin makes it easier for cells to absorb glucose from the bloodstream and use it as fuel, it is essential for controlling blood sugar levels. However, in individuals with Type 2 diabetes, cells become less responsive to insulin's actions, leading to impaired glucose uptake. This insulin resistance results in elevated levels of glucose in the bloodstream, a condition known as hyperglycemia.

Over time, the pancreas may struggle to keep up with the body's increased demand for insulin production, leading to relative insulin deficiency. This further contributes to elevated blood sugar levels, as the body's ability to regulate glucose becomes impaired.

Risk factors for Type 2 diabetes include obesity, physical inactivity, genetics, age, and certain ethnicities. Excess body weight, particularly abdominal fat, is strongly associated with insulin resistance and the development of Type 2 diabetes. Lack of regular physical activity can also increase the risk by promoting weight gain and exacerbating insulin resistance.

Symptoms of Type 2 diabetes may develop gradually and can include increased thirst and urination, fatigue, blurred vision, slow wound healing, and tingling or numbness in the hands or feet. However, some individuals with Type 2 diabetes may not experience any symptoms, especially in the early stages of the disease.

Diagnosis of Type 2 diabetes typically involves blood tests to measure fasting blood sugar levels, oral glucose tolerance tests, and hemoglobin A1c tests. Treatment aims to control blood sugar levels through lifestyle modifications, such as diet and exercise, oral medications, insulin therapy, and regular monitoring of blood sugar levels.

Understanding Type 2 diabetes is crucial for effective management and prevention of complications. By adopting a healthy lifestyle, monitoring blood sugar levels, and working closely with healthcare providers, individuals with Type 2 diabetes can lead fulfilling lives while minimizing the impact of the disease.

- Definition and Overview

Type 2 diabetes is a chronic metabolic disorder characterized by persistent high levels of blood sugar (glucose). Unlike Type 1 diabetes, which is an autoimmune condition where the body's immune system attacks and destroys insulin-producing cells in the pancreas, Type 2 diabetes typically develops due to a combination of genetic predisposition and lifestyle factors.

Overview of the Condition:

In Type 2 diabetes, the body either becomes resistant to the effects of insulin or does not produce enough insulin to maintain normal blood sugar levels. Insulin is a hormone produced by the pancreas that helps regulate glucose metabolism. It facilitates the uptake of glucose from the bloodstream into cells, where it is used for energy production.

Insulin Resistance:

In individuals with Type 2 diabetes, cells in the body become resistant to insulin's actions. This means that even though insulin is present, it is less effective at promoting glucose uptake into cells. High blood sugar levels are the result of glucose staying in the bloodstream.

Relative Insulin Deficiency:

In addition to insulin resistance, many people with Type 2 diabetes also experience relative insulin deficiency. This occurs when the pancreas cannot produce enough insulin to compensate for the body's increased demand.

Over time, the pancreas may lose its ability to produce insulin efficiently, exacerbating the problem.

Risk Factors:

The following are some of the factors that raise the risk of Type 2 diabetes:
- Obesity or excess body weight, particularly around the abdomen
- Sedentary behavior or a lack of exercise
- Genetics and family history of diabetes
- Age, with risk increasing after 45 years old
- Certain ethnicities, including African American, Hispanic/Latino, Native American, Asian American, and Pacific Islander

Symptoms:

Symptoms of Type 2 diabetes may include:
- Increased thirst and urination
- Fatigue
- Blurred vision
- Slow wound healing

- Tingling or numbness in the hands or feet

However, some individuals with Type 2 diabetes may not experience any symptoms, especially in the early stages of the disease.

Diagnosis and Treatment:
Diagnosis of Type 2 diabetes typically involves blood tests to measure fasting blood sugar levels, oral glucose tolerance tests, and hemoglobin A1c tests. Treatment focuses on controlling blood sugar levels through lifestyle modifications, such as diet and exercise, oral medications, insulin therapy, and regular monitoring of blood sugar levels.

Understanding the definition and overview of Type 2 diabetes is essential for recognizing the condition's signs, managing it effectively, and preventing complications. Early diagnosis and appropriate management can help individuals with Type 2 diabetes lead healthier lives and reduce the risk of long-term complications.

- How Type 2 Diabetes Differs from Type 1 Diabetes

Type 2 diabetes and Type 1 diabetes are both chronic conditions that affect the way the body regulates blood sugar (glucose), but they differ in several key aspects, including their causes, onset, and treatment.

1. Causes:

- Type 1 Diabetes: This autoimmune illness occurs when the immune system of the body unintentionally targets and kills the beta cells in the pancreas that produce insulin. Although the precise cause of this autoimmune reaction is not entirely known, environmental variables like virus infections and genetic predispositions may be involved.

- Type 2 Diabetes: Type 2 diabetes is primarily characterized by insulin resistance, where the body's cells become resistant to the effects of insulin, or relative insulin deficiency, where the The body cannot get enough insulin from the pancreas to meet its needs. While genetics also play a role in Type 2 diabetes, lifestyle factors such as obesity, physical inactivity, and poor diet are significant contributors to its development.

2. Onset:

- Type 1 Diabetes: Type 1 diabetes often develops in childhood or adolescence, although it can occur at any age. The onset is usually sudden, with symptoms appearing rapidly over a short period. Insulin therapy is necessary for lifelong survival for those with Type 1 diabetes.

- Type 2 Diabetes: Type 2 diabetes typically develops in adulthood, although it is increasingly being diagnosed in children and adolescents due to rising obesity rates. The onset of Type 2 diabetes is gradual, with symptoms often developing over several years. Initially, the pancreas may produce insulin, but the body's cells are resistant to its effects. Over time, insulin production may decrease, requiring additional interventions for management.

3. Treatment:

- Type 1 Diabetes: Treatment for Type 1 diabetes involves daily insulin injections or the use of an insulin pump to replace the insulin that the body no longer produces. Monitoring blood sugar levels, following a healthy diet, exercising regularly, and managing other health conditions are also essential components of Type 1 diabetes management.

- Type 2 Diabetes: Treatment for Type 2 diabetes focuses on lifestyle modifications, including dietary changes, regular physical activity, and weight management, to improve insulin sensitivity and blood sugar control. To assist lower blood sugar levels, doctors may prescribe oral drugs like metformin. In some cases, insulin therapy may also be necessary, particularly as the disease progresses.

4. Risk Factors:

- Type 1 Diabetes: Risk factors for Type 1 diabetes include family history, genetics, and certain environmental triggers, such as viral infections.

- Type 2 Diabetes: Risk factors for Type 2 diabetes include obesity, physical inactivity, genetics, age, ethnicity, and a history of gestational diabetes.

While Type 1 and Type 2 diabetes differ in their causes, onset, and treatment approaches, both conditions require lifelong management to prevent complications and maintain optimal health. Early diagnosis, education, and appropriate medical care are essential for individuals with either type of diabetes.

1.2 Causes and Risk Factors of Type 2 Diabetes

Type 2 diabetes is a complex condition influenced by a combination of genetic, environmental, and lifestyle factors. Understanding the causes and risk factors can help individuals assess their risk and take proactive steps to prevent or manage the condition effectively.

1. Genetic Factors:

- Family History: The likelihood of acquiring Type 2 diabetes is raised in cases when the disorder runs in the family. A person's genetic makeup greatly influences their likelihood of developing diabetes.

Certain gene variants may predispose individuals to insulin resistance or impair insulin production.

2. Lifestyle and Environmental Factors:

- Obesity: One of the biggest risk factors for Type 2 diabetes is being overweight, especially in the abdominal area. Adipose tissue, especially visceral fat, produces hormones and cytokines that contribute to insulin resistance and inflammation.

- Physical Inactivity: Sedentary lifestyles and lack of regular exercise are strongly associated with an increased risk of Type 2 diabetes. Physical activity helps improve insulin sensitivity, enhances glucose uptake by muscles, and promotes weight management.

- Unhealthy Diet: Diets high in refined carbohydrates, sugars, saturated fats, and processed foods contribute to obesity, insulin resistance, and elevated blood sugar levels. On the other hand, diets high in whole grains, fruits, vegetables, lean meats, and healthy fats can lower the risk of developing Type 2 diabetes.

- Gestational Diabetes: Pregnant women who acquire gestational diabetes are more likely to go on to acquire Type 2 diabetes in the future. Additionally, babies born to mothers with gestational diabetes may have a higher risk of developing obesity and Type 2 diabetes in adulthood.

3. Other Risk Factors:

- Age: Type 2 diabetes is more common as people age, especially after the age of 45. This may be due to age-related declines in insulin sensitivity and pancreatic function.

- Ethnicity: Certain ethnic groups, including African Americans, Hispanic/Latino Americans, Native Americans, Asian Americans, and Pacific Islanders, are at higher risk of developing Type 2 diabetes compared to Caucasians. These disparities may be influenced by genetic predisposition, cultural factors, and socioeconomic determinants of health.

- Medical Conditions: Certain medical conditions, such as polycystic ovary syndrome (PCOS), prediabetes, metabolic syndrome, and obstructive sleep apnea, increase the risk of developing Type 2 diabetes.

While some risk factors for Type 2 diabetes, such as genetics and age, cannot be modified, many lifestyle factors can be addressed to reduce the risk or delay the onset of the condition. Making healthy lifestyle choices, including maintaining a balanced diet, staying physically active, managing stress, and avoiding tobacco use, is crucial for diabetes prevention and overall well-being. Regular screening, early detection, and appropriate medical management are essential for individuals at risk or living with Type 2 diabetes to prevent complications and optimize health outcomes.

- Genetic Factors

Genetic factors play a significant role in the development of Type 2 diabetes, influencing an individual's susceptibility to the condition. While specific genetic variants associated with Type 2 diabetes have been identified, the inheritance pattern is complex, and multiple genes are involved. Here's a closer look at genetic factors contributing to Type 2 diabetes:

1. Family History:
   - Individuals with a family history of Type 2 diabetes are at increased risk of developing the condition

themselves. Having a parent or sibling with Type 2 diabetes can more than double an individual's risk compared to those with no family history. This suggests a strong genetic component in the development of the disease.

2. Genetic Variants:

 - Many genetic variations have been linked to Type 2 diabetes by genome-wide association studies (GWAS). These variants are involved in various biological pathways, including insulin production, insulin signaling, glucose metabolism, and pancreatic function.

 - One of the most well-known genetic variants associated with Type 2 diabetes is the TCF7L2 gene. Variants of this gene are strongly linked to an increased risk of Type 2 diabetes and impaired insulin secretion.

 - Other genes implicated in Type 2 diabetes include PPARG, KCNJ11, IRS1, and CAPN10, among others. These genes play roles in insulin sensitivity, pancreatic beta-cell function, and glucose homeostasis.

3. Epigenetics:

- Without changing the underlying DNA sequence, epigenetic alterations like DNA methylation and histone modifications can affect how genes are expressed. Epigenetic changes have been observed in individuals with Type 2 diabetes and may contribute to the development of insulin resistance and impaired glucose metabolism.

- Environmental factors, such as diet, physical activity, and exposure to toxins, can influence epigenetic modifications, potentially modulating an individual's risk of developing Type 2 diabetes.

4. Gene-Environment Interactions:

- Genetic predisposition to Type 2 diabetes interacts with environmental factors to determine an individual's overall risk. While genetic factors contribute to susceptibility, lifestyle factors such as diet, physical activity, obesity, and stress play crucial roles in triggering the onset of the disease.

- Individuals with a high genetic risk of Type 2 diabetes can mitigate their risk by adopting healthy lifestyle habits, while those with a lower genetic risk may still develop the condition if exposed to unfavorable environmental factors.

Understanding the role of genetic factors in Type 2 diabetes can help identify individuals at increased risk and inform personalized prevention and treatment strategies. While genetic predisposition contributes to susceptibility, lifestyle modifications remain paramount in managing and preventing Type 2 diabetes, emphasizing the importance of a holistic approach to health and wellness.

- Lifestyle and Environmental Factors

Lifestyle and environmental factors play a significant role in the development and progression of Type 2 diabetes. These modifiable factors, including diet, physical activity, obesity, and other lifestyle choices, interact with genetic predisposition to influence an individual's risk of developing the condition. Here's a closer look at how lifestyle and environmental factors contribute to Type 2 diabetes:

1. Diet:

- High Sugar and Refined Carbohydrate Intake:
Consuming a diet high in sugary beverages, processed
foods, and refined carbohydrates can lead to rapid
spikes in blood sugar levels, contributing to insulin
resistance and Type 2 diabetes.

- Low Fiber Intake: Diets low in fiber from fruits,
vegetables, and whole grains are associated with an
increased risk of Type 2 diabetes. Fiber helps regulate
blood sugar levels and promotes satiety, reducing the
risk of obesity and insulin resistance.

2. Physical Activity:

- Sedentary Lifestyle: Lack of regular physical activity
is a significant risk factor for Type 2 diabetes. Physical
inactivity contributes to weight gain, insulin resistance,
and impaired glucose metabolism. Regular exercise
helps improve insulin sensitivity, promotes weight loss,
and reduces the risk of developing Type 2 diabetes.

3. Obesity:

- Excess Body Weight: Obesity, particularly excess
abdominal fat, is strongly associated with an increased
risk of Type 2 diabetes. Adipose tissue, especially

visceral fat, produces hormones and cytokines that promote inflammation and insulin resistance. Losing weight through a combination of diet and exercise can improve insulin sensitivity and reduce the risk of Type 2 diabetes.

4. Smoking:

   - Tobacco Use: Smoking is a significant risk factor for Type 2 diabetes and can exacerbate existing diabetes-related complications. Tobacco smoke contains harmful chemicals that can impair insulin action and increase inflammation, contributing to insulin resistance and metabolic dysfunction.

5. Sleep Quality:

   - Sleep Disruption: Poor sleep quality, including insufficient sleep duration, irregular sleep patterns, and sleep disorders like obstructive sleep apnea, are associated with an increased risk of Type 2 diabetes. Sleep deprivation can disrupt hormonal regulation, leading to insulin resistance and glucose intolerance.

6. Environmental Exposures:

- Toxins and Pollutants: Exposure to environmental toxins, such as air pollution, heavy metals, and endocrine-disrupting chemicals, may contribute to the development of Type 2 diabetes. These toxins can interfere with insulin signaling pathways, disrupt glucose metabolism, and promote inflammation.

7. Socioeconomic Factors:

- Income and Education Level: Socioeconomic factors, including income level, education level, and access to healthcare services, influence an individual's risk of developing Type 2 diabetes. People with lower socioeconomic status are more likely to have limited access to healthy foods, safe neighborhoods for physical activity, and quality healthcare, increasing their risk of diabetes.

Addressing lifestyle and environmental factors through behavior modification, public health interventions, and policy changes is essential for preventing and managing Type 2 diabetes. Promoting healthy eating habits, encouraging regular physical activity, reducing tobacco use, improving sleep hygiene, and creating supportive environments can help reduce the burden of Type 2 diabetes and improve overall population health.

1.3 Recognizing the Symptoms

Recognizing the symptoms of Type 2 diabetes is crucial for early detection, diagnosis, and prompt intervention. While some individuals with Type 2 diabetes may experience symptoms gradually, others may not have noticeable symptoms at all, especially in the early stages of the disease. The following are typical indications and symptoms to be aware of:

1. Increased Thirst and Urination:
   - Experiencing frequent thirst (polydipsia) and urination (polyuria) is one of the hallmark symptoms of Type 2 diabetes. High blood sugar levels cause the kidneys to work harder to filter and absorb excess glucose, leading to increased urine production and dehydration.

2. Fatigue and Weakness:

  - Persistent fatigue, weakness, and feelings of exhaustion can be symptoms of uncontrolled Type 2 diabetes. Insulin resistance and impaired glucose metabolism can disrupt the body's ability to use glucose for energy, leading to feelings of tiredness and lethargy. distorted vision may occur when high blood sugar levels cause fluid to be pulled from the lenses of the eyes, affecting their ability to focus properly. This symptom is usually temporary and may improve with better blood sugar control.

3. Blurred Vision:

  - Blurred or of Type 2 diabetes. Insulin resistance and impaired glucose metabolism can prevent the body from properly using calories for energy, leading to unintentional weight loss.

4. Slow Wound Healing:

- The body's capacity to recover wounds and injuries may be hampered by type 2 diabetes. High blood sugar levels can damage blood vessels and nerves, leading to poor circulation and reduced immune function. As a result, cuts, bruises, and other wounds may take longer to heal and be more prone to infections.

5. Recurrent Infections:
  - People with Type 2 diabetes may be more susceptible to infections, including urinary tract infections, skin infections, and yeast infections. High blood sugar levels create an ideal environment for bacteria and fungi to thrive, increasing the risk of infections.

6. Tingling or Numbness:
  - Nerve damage (neuropathy) caused by prolonged exposure to high blood sugar levels can lead to tingling, numbness, or burning sensations in the hands, feet, or legs. This symptom, known as diabetic neuropathy, typically develops over time and may worsen if diabetes is not well-controlled.

7. Unexplained Weight Loss:

- Unexpected weight loss, despite maintaining normal eating habits or even increased appetite, can be a sign

8. Other Symptoms:

- Other symptoms of Type 2 diabetes may include increased hunger (polyphagia), dry mouth, itchy skin, and dark patches of skin (acanthosis nigricans) in areas such as the neck, armpits, or groin. It's important to note that not everyone with Type 2 diabetes will experience all of these symptoms, and some individuals may not have any symptoms at all. Additionally, symptoms may vary in severity from person to person. To ensure a correct examination and diagnosis, it is imperative that you visit a healthcare expert if you encounter any of these symptoms or have concerns regarding your health. Type 2 diabetes can be prevented from developing complications and have better long-term health outcomes with early detection and control.

- Common Symptoms

Common symptoms of Type 2 diabetes can vary from person to person and may develop gradually over time. Some individuals may not experience any symptoms, especially in the early stages of the disease. However, recognizing the following common symptoms can prompt early detection and intervention:

1. Increased Thirst and Urination (Polydipsia and Polyuria):
  - Feeling unusually thirsty and needing to urinate more frequently than usual are common symptoms of Type 2 diabetes. High blood sugar levels cause the kidneys to work harder to filter and absorb glucose, leading to increased urine production and dehydration.

2. Fatigue and Weakness:
  - Persistent fatigue, weakness, and feelings of exhaustion can be early signs of Type 2 diabetes. Insulin resistance and impaired glucose metabolism can disrupt the body's ability to use glucose for energy, leading to feelings of tiredness and lethargy.

3. Blurred Vision:

- Blurred or distorted vision may occur when high blood sugar levels affect the lenses of the eyes, leading to changes in vision. This symptom is usually temporary and may improve with better blood sugar control.

4. Slow Wound Healing:

- The body's capacity to recover wounds and injuries may be hampered by type 2 diabetes. High blood sugar levels can damage blood vessels and nerves, leading to poor circulation and reduced immune function. As a result, cuts, bruises, and other wounds may take longer to heal and be more prone to infections.

5. Recurrent Infections:

- People with Type 2 diabetes may experience more frequent infections, including urinary tract infections, skin infections, and yeast infections. High blood sugar levels create an ideal environment for bacteria and fungi to thrive, increasing the risk of infections.

6. Hand or foot tingling or numbness:

- Nerve damage (neuropathy) caused by prolonged exposure to high blood sugar levels can lead to tingling, numbness, or burning sensations in the hands, feet, or legs. This symptom, known as diabetic neuropathy, typically develops over time and may worsen if diabetes is not well-controlled.

7. Unexplained Weight Loss:
  - Unexpected weight loss, despite maintaining normal eating habits or even increased appetite, can be a sign of Type 2 diabetes. Insulin resistance and impaired glucose metabolism can prevent the body from properly using calories for energy, leading to unintentional weight loss.

8. Other Symptoms:
  - Additional symptoms of Type 2 diabetes may include increased hunger (polyphagia), dry mouth, itchy skin, and dark patches of skin (acanthosis nigricans) in areas such as the neck, armpits, or groin.

If you experience any of these symptoms or have concerns about your health, it's important to consult with a healthcare professional for proper evaluation and diagnosis. Type 2 diabetes can be prevented from developing complications and have better long-term health outcomes with early detection and control.

- When to See a Doctor

It's important to see a doctor if you experience any signs or symptoms of Type 2 diabetes or if you have risk factors for the condition. Here are some situations when you should consider seeking medical attention:

1. Presence of Symptoms: If you experience symptoms such as increased thirst, frequent urination, unexplained weight loss, fatigue, blurred vision, slow wound healing, tingling or numbness in the hands or feet, or recurrent infections, it's essential to consult with a healthcare professional. These symptoms may indicate underlying health issues, including Type 2 diabetes, that require evaluation and management.

2. Risk Factors: If you have risk factors for Type 2 diabetes, such as being overweight or obese, having a family history of diabetes, being physically inactive, or having other medical conditions such as high blood pressure or high cholesterol, you should consider

discussing your risk with a doctor. Early detection and intervention can help prevent or delay the onset of Type 2 diabetes and its complications.

3. **Routine Screening:** Even if you don't have symptoms or risk factors, it's recommended to undergo routine screening for Type 2 diabetes, especially if you are over 45 years old or belong to high-risk ethnic groups. Screening tests, such as fasting blood sugar tests, oral glucose tolerance tests, or hemoglobin A1c tests, can help detect diabetes early when treatment is most effective.

4. Gestational Diabetes: If you are pregnant or planning to become pregnant, it's important to undergo screening for gestational diabetes, a type of diabetes that develops during pregnancy. Women with gestational diabetes have an increased risk of developing Type 2 diabetes later in life and should receive appropriate medical care and monitoring.

5. Follow-Up Care: If you have already been diagnosed with Type 2 diabetes, it's crucial to attend regular

follow-up appointments with your healthcare provider to monitor your condition, adjust treatment as needed, and prevent complications. Your doctor can help you develop a personalized diabetes management plan that includes lifestyle modifications, medications, blood sugar monitoring, and other interventions to optimize your health and well-being.

Overall, if you have any concerns about your health or suspect that you may have Type 2 diabetes, don't hesitate to schedule an appointment with a doctor or healthcare provider. Early detection, proper diagnosis, and timely intervention are key to effectively managing Type 2 diabetes and reducing the risk of complications.

1.4 Getting Diagnosed

Getting diagnosed with Type 2 diabetes involves several steps, including screening, testing, and evaluation by a healthcare professional. Here's an overview of the process:

1. Risk Assessment:

  - Before undergoing diagnostic tests, your doctor will assess your risk factors for Type 2 diabetes. This may include evaluating your age, family history, medical history, lifestyle factors (such as diet and physical activity), and any symptoms you may be experiencing.

2. Screening Tests:

  - If you are at increased risk or show symptoms of Type 2 diabetes, your doctor may recommend screening tests to assess your blood sugar levels. Common screening tests include:

  - Fasting Plasma Glucose Test: After at least eight hours of fasting, this test determines your blood sugar level. To measure the levels of fasting blood sugar, a blood sample is obtained. A blood sugar level after fasting of 126 milligrams per deciliter (mg/dL) or higher indicates diabetes.

  - Oral Glucose Tolerance Test (OGTT): This test involves drinking a sugary solution, and blood sugar levels are measured before and two hours after drinking the solution. Diabetes is indicated by a blood sugar level of 200 mg/dL or above two hours after consuming the solution.

- Hemoglobin A1c Test: This examination calculates your blood sugar average for the previous two to three months. An A1c level of 6.5% or higher indicates diabetes.

3. Diagnosis Confirmation:
  - If the results of your screening tests indicate diabetes, your doctor may perform additional tests to confirm the diagnosis and determine the type of diabetes you have. These tests may include repeating the screening tests on a different day or conducting further laboratory tests.

4. Evaluation and Treatment Planning:
  - Once the diagnosis of Type 2 diabetes is confirmed, your doctor will discuss the implications of the diagnosis with you and develop a personalized treatment plan. This plan may include lifestyle modifications (such as diet and exercise), medications (such as oral antidiabetic drugs), blood sugar monitoring, and regular follow-up appointments.

5. Education and Support:

   - After diagnosis, your healthcare team will provide you with education and support to help you manage your diabetes effectively. This may include information on blood sugar monitoring, meal planning, medication management, exercise recommendations, and strategies for preventing complications. Diabetes education programs and support groups may also be available to help you navigate life with diabetes.

Overall, getting diagnosed with Type 2 diabetes is the first step toward effectively managing the condition and preventing complications. By working closely with your healthcare team and following your treatment plan, you can take control of your diabetes and lead a healthy, fulfilling life.

   - **Medical Tests and Diagnosis**

Medical tests and diagnosis of Type 2 diabetes involve several steps to assess blood sugar levels, confirm the diagnosis, and determine the appropriate course of treatment. Here's an overview of the medical tests and diagnostic process:

1. Initial Assessment:
   - Your healthcare provider will begin by evaluating your medical history, risk factors, and symptoms associated with Type 2 diabetes. Factors such as family history of diabetes, age, ethnicity, obesity, sedentary lifestyle, and gestational diabetes history may increase your risk and warrant further testing.

2. Screening Tests:
   - Screening tests are used to assess blood sugar levels and identify individuals at risk or suspected of having Type 2 diabetes. Common screening tests include:
   - Fasting Plasma Glucose Test: This test measures blood sugar levels after fasting for at least eight hours. A fasting blood sugar level of 126 milligrams per deciliter (mg/dL) or higher on two separate occasions is diagnostic of diabetes.
   - Oral Glucose Tolerance Test (OGTT): After fasting, you drink a sugary solution, and blood sugar levels are

measured before and two hours after drinking it. A blood sugar level of 200 mg/dL or higher two hours after the drink confirms diabetes.

-A1c test for hemoglobin: This test calculates the mean blood sugar levels throughout the previous two to three months. An A1c level of 6.5% or higher indicates diabetes.

3. Confirmation of Diagnosis:

- If initial screening tests indicate diabetes, your healthcare provider may repeat the tests on a different day to confirm the diagnosis. This helps rule out temporary fluctuations in blood sugar levels or lab errors.

- In some cases, additional tests may be performed to differentiate between Type 1 and Type 2 diabetes, such as measuring levels of pancreatic autoantibodies or assessing insulin production and sensitivity.

4. Comprehensive Evaluation:

- Once the diagnosis of Type 2 diabetes is confirmed, your healthcare provider may conduct a comprehensive evaluation to assess your overall health, including a physical examination, laboratory tests (such as lipid profile, kidney function tests, and liver function tests), and assessment of diabetes-related complications.

5. Treatment Planning:
  - Based on the results of diagnostic tests and evaluation, your healthcare provider will develop a personalized treatment plan tailored to your needs. This may include lifestyle modifications (such as diet and exercise), oral medications (such as metformin), insulin therapy, blood sugar monitoring, and regular follow-up appointments.

6. Ongoing Monitoring and Management:
  - After diagnosis, ongoing monitoring and management are essential to control blood sugar levels, prevent complications, and optimize overall health. This may involve regular blood sugar monitoring, medication adjustments, lifestyle counseling, and periodic evaluations of diabetes-related complications.

Overall, early detection and diagnosis of Type 2 diabetes are crucial for initiating timely treatment and preventing complications. By working closely with your healthcare team and following your treatment plan, you can effectively manage your diabetes and lead a healthy, fulfilling life.

- Understanding Your Diagnosis

Understanding your diagnosis of Type 2 diabetes is essential for effectively managing the condition and optimizing your health outcomes. Here's a comprehensive guide to help you understand your diagnosis:

1. Explanation of Type 2 Diabetes:
   - Your healthcare provider will explain that Type 2 diabetes is a chronic condition characterized by elevated blood sugar levels due to insulin resistance and/or impaired insulin production by the pancreas. They may describe how insulin normally helps regulate blood sugar levels and how dysfunction in this process leads to diabetes.

2. Discussion of Diagnostic Tests:

  - Your healthcare provider will review the results of the diagnostic tests used to confirm your diagnosis, such as fasting plasma glucose, oral glucose tolerance test (OGTT), or hemoglobin A1c test. They will explain what each test measures and how the results indicate the presence of diabetes.

3. Risk Factors and Contributing Factors:

  - Your healthcare provider may discuss the risk factors and contributing factors that predisposed you to developing Type 2 diabetes. This may include factors such as family history, obesity, sedentary lifestyle, unhealthy diet, age, ethnicity, and history of gestational diabetes.

4. Symptoms and Signs:

  - If you experienced symptoms or signs of diabetes before diagnosis, your healthcare provider will discuss them with you and explain how they relate to the condition. Increased thirst, frequent urination, unexplained weight loss, exhaustion, hazy eyesight, and sluggish wound healing are typical symptoms.

5. Importance of Treatment and Management:
  - Your healthcare provider will emphasize the importance of treatment and management to control blood sugar levels, prevent complications, and improve your quality of life. They will explain that Type 2 diabetes requires ongoing management and that successful treatment often involves a combination of lifestyle modifications, medications, and regular monitoring.

6. Treatment Options:
  - Your healthcare provider will discuss treatment options available for Type 2 diabetes and help you develop a personalized treatment plan based on your individual needs, preferences, and health goals. This may include lifestyle modifications (such as diet, exercise, and weight management), oral medications (such as metformin or sulfonylureas), insulin therapy, and other interventions.

7. Education and Support:

   - Your healthcare provider may provide educational resources, counseling, and support to help you understand and manage your diabetes effectively. This may include information on blood sugar monitoring, meal planning, medication management, exercise recommendations, and strategies for preventing complications.

8. Follow-Up Care:

   - Your healthcare provider will schedule regular follow-up appointments to monitor your progress, adjust your treatment plan as needed, and address any concerns or questions you may have. They will emphasize the importance of ongoing monitoring, adherence to treatment, and proactive management to achieve optimal outcomes.

Understanding your diagnosis of Type 2 diabetes empowers you to take control of your health and actively participate in your treatment and management. By working closely with your healthcare team, making informed decisions, and adopting healthy lifestyle habits, you can effectively manage your diabetes and live a fulfilling life.

Chapter 2:

- Managing Your Diabetes

Managing diabetes involves a comprehensive approach that includes diet, exercise, medication (if prescribed), regular monitoring of blood sugar levels, and maintaining a healthy lifestyle overall. Here's a breakdown of key aspects:

1. Healthy Eating: Focus on a balanced diet rich in fruits, vegetables, lean proteins, and whole grains. Limit processed foods, sugary drinks, and excessive carbohydrates. Blood sugar levels can be stabilized by distributing meals throughout the day and keeping an eye on portion amounts.

2. Regular Exercise: As it improves insulin sensitivity, lowers blood sugar, and helps regulate weight, physical activity is essential for managing diabetes. In addition to strength training activities, try to get in at least 150 minutes a week of moderate aerobic activity or 75 minutes of intense activity.

3. Medication Adherence: If prescribed, take your medication as directed by your healthcare provider. This may include insulin injections, oral medications, or other treatments to help regulate blood sugar levels.

4. Blood Sugar Monitoring: Regularly check your blood sugar levels as advised by your healthcare provider. This helps you understand how your body responds to food, exercise, medication, and other factors, allowing you to make necessary adjustments.

5. Stress Management: Stress can affect blood sugar levels, so incorporating stress-reducing techniques such as meditation, deep breathing exercises, or hobbies can be beneficial.

6. Regular Medical Checkups: Attend regular checkups with your healthcare team to monitor your diabetes management, adjust treatment plans if needed, and address any concerns or complications.

7. Foot Care: Diabetes can lead to nerve damage and poor circulation, increasing the risk of foot problems. Check your feet daily for any cuts, sores, or blisters, and seek prompt medical attention for any issues.

8. Quit Smoking: Smoking can worsen diabetes complications, so if you smoke, seek support to quit.

9. Stay Informed: Educate yourself about diabetes and its management. Understand how different foods, activities, and medications affect your body, and stay updated on the latest research and recommendations.

10. Support System: Surround yourself with supportive friends, family, or diabetes support groups who understand your challenges and can provide encouragement and assistance when needed.

Remember, managing diabetes is a lifelong commitment, but with dedication and support, you can lead a full and healthy life.

2.1 Monitoring Blood Sugar Levels

One of the most important parts of properly managing diabetes is blood sugar monitoring. Here's what you need to know about monitoring:

1. Frequency: The frequency of monitoring may vary depending on the type of diabetes, treatment plan, and individual circumstances. Some people may need to check their blood sugar multiple times a day, while others may require less frequent monitoring.

2. Timing: It's essential to monitor blood sugar levels at specific times, such as before meals, after meals, before and after exercise, before bedtime, and if you suspect low blood sugar (hypoglycemia) symptoms.

3. Methods: There are several methods for monitoring blood sugar levels, including:

 - Blood Glucose Meters: These handheld devices measure blood sugar levels using a small drop of blood obtained by pricking the fingertip with a lancet. Results are available within seconds.

   - Continuous Glucose Monitoring (CGM) Systems: CGM systems use a sensor inserted under the skin to measure glucose levels in the interstitial fluid. They provide real-time glucose readings throughout the day and night, offering insights into trends and patterns.

4. Target Range: Your healthcare provider will establish target blood sugar ranges for you based on factors such as age, type of diabetes, overall health, and treatment plan. Aim to keep your blood sugar levels within these target ranges to reduce the risk of complications.

5. Interpreting Results: Understand what your blood sugar readings mean and how they relate to your overall diabetes management. Regularly review your blood sugar logs with your healthcare team to identify trends, make adjustments to your treatment plan, and address any concerns.

6. Record Keeping: Keep a record of your blood sugar readings, along with details such as meals, medications, exercise, and any symptoms or factors that may affect blood sugar levels. Together with your healthcare professional, you may use this information to make well-informed decisions regarding the management of your diabetes.

7. Response to Readings: Know how to respond to high or low blood sugar levels based on your healthcare provider's recommendations. This may include adjusting your insulin dose, eating a snack, drinking juice or glucose tablets for low blood sugar, or seeking medical attention if necessary.

8. Calibration and Maintenance: Ensure that your blood glucose meter or CGM system is calibrated correctly and maintained according to the manufacturer's instructions to ensure accurate results.

By monitoring your blood sugar levels regularly and understanding the significance of the results, you can take proactive steps to manage your diabetes effectively and minimize the risk of complications.

- How to Monitor

Monitoring blood sugar levels involves several steps. Here's a guide on how to monitor your blood sugar effectively:

1. Choose a Monitoring Method: Decide whether you'll use a traditional blood glucose meter or a continuous glucose monitoring (CGM) system based on your healthcare provider's recommendations, your lifestyle, and your preferences.

2. Prepare the Equipment: If you're using a blood glucose meter, ensure you have all the necessary supplies: a blood glucose meter, test strips, lancet device, lancets, and alcohol swabs. If you're using a CGM system, ensure the sensor is properly inserted and connected to the receiver or smartphone app.

3. Wash Your Hands: Before testing your blood sugar, wash your hands thoroughly with soap and water and

dry them completely. This helps ensure accurate results by removing any dirt, oils, or residue from your skin.

4. Prepare the Testing Site: If you're using a blood glucose meter, choose a fingertip for testing. Use the lancet device to prick the side of your fingertip (avoiding the center) to obtain a small drop of blood. If you're using a CGM system, follow the manufacturer's instructions for sensor placement and insertion.

5. Perform the Test: If you're using a blood glucose meter, insert a test strip into the meter and apply the blood sample to the test strip. Await the blood sugar reading on the meter to appear. If you're using a CGM system, check the receiver or smartphone app for real-time glucose readings.

6. Record the Results: Write down or enter the blood sugar reading into a logbook, smartphone app, or digital spreadsheet along with details such as the date, time, pre-meal or post-meal status, medications, exercise, and any symptoms or factors that may have affected the result.

7. Interpret the Results: Compare your blood sugar reading to your target range and consider factors such as recent meals, medications, physical activity, and stress levels. Note any patterns or trends in your blood sugar levels over time.

8. Take Action if Necessary: If your blood sugar is outside your target range, follow your healthcare provider's recommendations for adjusting your treatment plan. This may involve adjusting your insulin dose, eating a snack, drinking juice or glucose tablets for low blood sugar, or seeking medical attention if necessary.

9. Maintain Consistency: Monitor your blood sugar levels consistently according to your healthcare provider's recommendations and incorporate the results into your diabetes management plan.

10. Regularly Review with Your Healthcare Team: Share your blood sugar logs and any concerns or questions with your healthcare provider and diabetes care team

during regular checkups to evaluate your progress and, if necessary, modify your treatment strategy.

By following these steps and maintaining a regular monitoring routine, you can effectively manage your blood sugar levels and take control of your diabetes.

- **Understanding Blood Sugar Readings**

Understanding blood sugar readings is essential for effectively managing diabetes. Here's how to interpret blood sugar readings:

1. Normal Range: For most individuals, blood sugar levels typically range between 70 to 99 milligrams per deciliter (mg/dL) when fasting (before meals) and less than 140 mg/dL two hours after eating. However, target ranges may vary depending on individual factors and treatment goals.

2. Fasting Blood Sugar (FBS): This measures blood sugar levels after an overnight fast (usually eight hours). A fasting blood sugar level below 100 mg/dL is generally considered normal. Levels between 100 to 125 mg/dL

may indicate prediabetes, while levels of 126 mg/dL or higher on two separate tests may indicate diabetes.

3. Postprandial Blood Sugar: This measures blood sugar levels one to two hours after eating. A postprandial blood sugar level below 140 mg/dL is considered normal for most individuals. However, people with diabetes may have different target ranges depending on their treatment plan and individual circumstances.

4. Random Blood Sugar: This measures blood sugar levels at any time of the day, regardless of when you last ate. Random blood sugar levels below 200 mg/dL are generally considered normal. However, if levels consistently exceed this threshold, it may indicate diabetes or other health concerns.

5. Hemoglobin A1c (HbA1c): Your average blood sugar levels over the previous two to three months are determined by this blood test. The outcomes are expressed as a percentage, whereby lower percentages signify improved regulation of blood sugar. For most people, a target HbA1c level is below 7%, although

individual targets may vary based on age, health status, and other factors.

6. Interpreting High Blood Sugar (Hyperglycemia): High blood sugar levels (hyperglycemia) can occur for various reasons, including inadequate insulin dosing, missed medications, excessive carbohydrate intake, illness, stress, or lack of physical activity. Increased thirst, frequent urination, exhaustion, impaired eyesight, and sluggish wound healing are possible symptoms. If your blood sugar levels consistently exceed your target range, consult your healthcare provider to adjust your treatment plan.

7. Interpreting Low Blood Sugar (Hypoglycemia): Low blood sugar levels (hypoglycemia) occur when blood sugar levels drop below normal (typically below 70 mg/dL). This can result from too much insulin or diabetes medication, delayed or missed meals, excessive exercise, or alcohol consumption. Symptoms may include shakiness, sweating, irritability, confusion, weakness, and dizziness. If you experience hypoglycemia, consume a fast-acting carbohydrate such

as glucose tablets, juice, or candy to raise your blood sugar levels promptly.

8. Pattern Recognition: Regularly monitor your blood sugar levels and track patterns and trends over time. Look for consistent highs or lows at certain times of the day, which can help identify factors contributing to fluctuations in blood sugar levels and inform adjustments to your diabetes management plan.

By understanding your blood sugar readings and their implications, you can make informed decisions to manage your diabetes effectively and minimize the risk of complications. Regular communication with your healthcare provider is essential for setting appropriate blood sugar targets and developing a personalized treatment plan.

2.2 Medication and Insulin Therapy

Medication and insulin therapy are essential components of managing diabetes, particularly for individuals with type 1 diabetes or type 2 diabetes who require additional support in controlling blood sugar levels. Here's an overview:

1. Oral Medications (for Type 2 Diabetes):
   - Metformin: Often the first-line medication for type 2 diabetes, metformin helps lower blood sugar levels by reducing glucose production in the liver and improving insulin sensitivity in the muscles.
   - Sulfonylureas: These medications stimulate the pancreas to produce more insulin, helping lower blood sugar levels. Examples include glipizide, glyburide, and glimepiride.
   - DPP-4 Inhibitors: These drugs increase insulin production and decrease glucose production in the liver. Examples include sitagliptin, saxagliptin, and linagliptin.
   - SGLT2 Inhibitors: These drugs cause the kidneys to excrete sugar from the body through urine, which lowers blood sugar levels. Examples include canagliflozin, dapagliflozin, and empagliflozin.
   - GLP-1 Receptor Agonists: These injectable medications help lower blood sugar levels by increasing

insulin secretion, slowing gastric emptying, and reducing appetite. Examples include liraglutide, dulaglutide, and exenatide.

2. Insulin Therapy (for Type 1 and Type 2 Diabetes):

- Rapid-Acting Insulin: This type of insulin begins to work within 15 minutes after injection and peaks in about 1 to 2 hours. It's typically taken just before or with meals to help control blood sugar levels after eating.

- Short-Acting Insulin: Short-acting insulin starts working within 30 minutes after injection and peaks in 2 to 3 hours. It's often used to cover blood sugar increases from meals and may be taken before meals.

- Intermediate-Acting Insulin: This type of insulin takes longer to start working (about 2 to 4 hours) but lasts longer, with peak action occurring in 4 to 12 hours. It's usually taken twice daily to provide basal insulin coverage between meals and overnight.

- Long-Acting Insulin: Long-acting insulin provides a steady level of insulin throughout the day and night, with no pronounced peaks. It's taken once or twice daily to provide basal insulin coverage and maintain stable blood sugar levels between meals and overnight.

- Premixed Insulin: These insulin formulations combine rapid- or short-acting insulin with intermediate-acting insulin in fixed ratios. They're often used to simplify insulin regimens and provide both basal and mealtime insulin coverage.

3. Insulin Delivery Methods:
  - Insulin Pens: These disposable devices contain pre-filled insulin cartridges and are used to inject insulin.
  - Insulin Syringes: These are used to draw insulin from vials and inject it into the body.
  - Insulin Pumps: These devices continuously deliver insulin through a small tube inserted under the skin. They can provide more precise insulin dosing and flexibility in managing blood sugar levels.

4. Monitoring and Adjusting Therapy:
  - Regularly monitor blood sugar levels to assess the effectiveness of medication and insulin therapy.
  - Work closely with your healthcare provider to adjust medication doses, timing, and delivery methods based on blood sugar readings, lifestyle factors, and individual needs.

- Follow your healthcare provider's guidance on insulin dosing adjustments for meals, physical activity, illness, and other factors that may affect blood sugar levels.

Medication and insulin therapy play a crucial role in managing diabetes and achieving target blood sugar levels. It's essential to work closely with your healthcare provider to develop a personalized treatment plan that meets your needs and helps you maintain optimal health and well-being.

- **Types of Medications**

Medications for diabetes can be categorized based on their mechanism of action and how they help manage blood sugar levels. Here are the main types:

1. Biguanides:
- Metformin: It's the most commonly prescribed medication for type 2 diabetes. Metformin works by reducing glucose production in the liver and increasing

insulin sensitivity in the muscles, leading to lower blood sugar levels.

2. Sulfonylureas:
   - These medications stimulate the pancreas to produce more insulin, helping lower blood sugar levels.
   - Examples include glipizide, glyburide, and glimepiride.

3. Meglitinides:
   - Similar to sulfonylureas, meglitinides also stimulate insulin secretion from the pancreas.
   - Examples include repaglinide and nateglinide.

4. DPP-4 Inhibitors (Dipeptidyl Peptidase-4 Inhibitors):
   - These medications increase insulin production and decrease glucose production in the liver.
   - Saxagliptin, linagliptin, alogliptin, and sitagliptin are a few examples.

5. SGLT2 Inhibitors (Sodium-Glucose Cotransporter-2 Inhibitors):

- SGLT2 inhibitors lower blood sugar levels by causing the kidneys to remove sugar from the body through urine.
   - Examples include canagliflozin, dapagliflozin, and empagliflozin.

6. GLP-1 Receptor Agonists (Glucagon-Like Peptide-1 Receptor Agonists):
   - These injectable medications increase insulin secretion, slow gastric emptying, and reduce appetite.
   - Examples include liraglutide, dulaglutide, exenatide, and semaglutide.

7. Thiazolidinediones (TZDs):
   - TZDs help improve insulin sensitivity in the body's cells, reducing blood sugar levels.
   - Examples include pioglitazone and rosiglitazone.

8. Alpha-Glucosidase Inhibitors:
   - These medications slow down the digestion of carbohydrates in the intestines, helping to reduce blood sugar spikes after meals.
   - Examples include acarbose and miglitol.

9. Combination Therapies:
  - Some medications combine two or more types of
diabetes drugs to provide complementary mechanisms
of action and improve blood sugar control.
  - Examples include combinations of metformin with
sulfonylureas, DPP-4 inhibitors, or SGLT2 inhibitors.

10. Insulin:
  Insulin is a hormone that promotes the uptake of
glucose into cells, which helps control blood sugar
levels.
  - Types of insulin include rapid-acting, short-acting,
intermediate-acting, and long-acting insulin, as well as
premixed insulin formulations.

Each type of medication works in a different way to help
manage blood sugar levels. Your healthcare provider
will consider factors such as your type of diabetes,
overall health, other medical conditions, and individual
treatment goals when prescribing medication therapy.
It's essential to follow your healthcare provider's

recommendations and regularly monitor your blood sugar levels to ensure effective diabetes management.

- How Insulin Works and How to Use It

Insulin is a hormone produced by the pancreas that plays a crucial role in regulating blood sugar levels. Here's how insulin works and how to use it:

How Insulin Works:

1. Glucose Uptake: When you eat carbohydrates, your digestive system breaks them down into glucose, a type of sugar that enters the bloodstream. In response to rising blood sugar levels, the pancreas releases insulin into the bloodstream.

2. Cellular Uptake: Insulin acts as a "key" that allows glucose to enter cells throughout the body, where it's used for energy. Insulin binds to receptors on the surface of cells, triggering the uptake of glucose from the bloodstream into the cells.

3. Liver Regulation: Insulin also helps regulate glucose production in the liver. It suppresses the liver's release of glucose into the bloodstream and promotes the storage of excess glucose in the form of glycogen.

4. Fat Storage: Insulin promotes the storage of excess glucose as fat in adipose tissue, helping to maintain energy balance in the body.

5. Protein Synthesis: Insulin facilitates the uptake of amino acids into cells and promotes protein synthesis, supporting tissue growth and repair.

How to Use Insulin:

1. Selecting the Right Insulin: There are different types of insulin available, including rapid-acting, short-acting, intermediate-acting, and long-acting insulin formulations. Your healthcare provider will prescribe the type(s) of insulin that best meet your individual needs based on factors such as your type of diabetes, blood sugar control goals, lifestyle, and preferences.

2. Insulin Delivery Methods:

   - Insulin Pens: These pens are practical and simple to use. They contain pre-filled insulin cartridges and have a dial to select the desired dose. Insulin pens are available for rapid-acting, short-acting, and long-acting insulin.

   - Insulin Syringes**: Insulin syringes are used to draw insulin from vials and inject it into the body. They come in different sizes and have markings to measure the dose accurately.

   - Insulin Pumps: Insulin pumps deliver insulin continuously through a small tube inserted under the skin. They allow for precise insulin dosing and flexibility in managing blood sugar levels.

3. Injection Technique:

   - Choose the Injection Site: Common injection sites include the abdomen, thighs, buttocks, and upper arms. Rotate injection sites within the same area to prevent lipodystrophy (changes in fat tissue).

   - Clean the Injection Site: Wash your hands and the injection site with soap and water. Allow the skin to dry before injecting insulin.

- Prepare the Insulin: If using a vial and syringe, draw the correct dose of insulin into the syringe. If using an insulin pen, set the dose according to your healthcare provider's instructions.

- Inject the Insulin: Insert the needle into the skin at a 90-degree angle (or as directed) and inject the insulin. Press the plunger all the way down to deliver the full dose. Hold the needle in place for a few seconds before withdrawing it to ensure all the insulin is delivered.

4. Dosage and Timing: Follow your healthcare provider's instructions regarding insulin dosage, timing, and frequency of administration. Insulin doses may vary based on factors such as meal size, carbohydrate intake, physical activity, and blood sugar levels.

5. Monitoring and Adjustments: Regularly monitor your blood sugar levels and adjust insulin doses as needed based on your healthcare provider's recommendations. Keep track of your insulin injections, blood sugar readings, meals, and physical activity to help fine-tune your insulin regimen.

6. Storage: Store insulin according to the manufacturer's instructions, typically in the refrigerator until opened and at room temperature once opened. Avoid exposure to extreme temperatures, direct sunlight, and freezing.

7. Safety Precautions: Always use clean injection equipment, rotate injection sites, and follow proper hygiene practices to reduce the risk of infection. Dispose of needles and syringes safely in puncture-proof containers.

8. Consult Your Healthcare Provider: If you have any questions or concerns about using insulin, consult your healthcare provider or diabetes care team for guidance and support.

By understanding how insulin works and following proper techniques for insulin use, you can effectively manage your diabetes and achieve target blood sugar levels. Regular communication with your healthcare provider is essential for optimizing insulin therapy and maintaining optimal health and well-being.

2.3 Diet and Nutrition

Diet and nutrition play a fundamental role in managing diabetes effectively. Here are some essential ideas to think about:

1. Balanced Meals: Aim for balanced meals that include a variety of nutrient-rich foods from all food groups: fruits, vegetables, lean proteins, whole grains, and healthy fats. This helps provide essential nutrients while controlling blood sugar levels.

2. Carbohydrate Management: Carbohydrates have the most significant impact on blood sugar levels. Focus on choosing complex carbohydrates with a low glycemic index (GI), such as whole grains, legumes, fruits, and vegetables, which are digested more slowly and cause gradual increases in blood sugar levels. Monitor portion sizes and distribute carbohydrates evenly throughout the day to help manage blood sugar levels effectively.

3. Healthy Fats: Include sources of healthy fats in your diet, such as avocados, nuts, seeds, olive oil, and fatty

fish like salmon and mackerel. Heart health and insulin sensitivity are enhanced by heart-healthy lipids.

4. Lean Proteins: Incorporate lean protein sources into your meals, such as poultry, fish, tofu, beans, lentils, and low-fat dairy products. Protein encourages fullness and aids in blood sugar stabilization.

5. Fiber-Rich Foods: Choose fiber-rich foods, including fruits, vegetables, whole grains, legumes, and nuts, which can help regulate blood sugar levels, improve digestion, and support weight management.

6. Meal Timing and Spacing: Eat regular meals and snacks throughout the day to maintain consistent energy levels and prevent spikes or drops in blood sugar. Aim to space meals evenly and avoid prolonged periods of fasting.

7. Portion Control: Pay attention to portion sizes to avoid overeating, which can lead to spikes in blood sugar levels. Use measuring cups, food scales, or visual

cues to help control portion sizes, especially for carbohydrate-containing foods.

8. Hydration: Stay hydrated by drinking plenty of water throughout the day. Limit sugary drinks and alcohol, which can contribute to spikes in blood sugar levels and interfere with diabetes management.

9. Limit Added Sugars and Processed Foods: Minimize your intake of foods and beverages high in added sugars, refined carbohydrates, and processed ingredients. These can cause rapid increases in blood sugar levels and contribute to weight gain and other health issues.

10. Monitor Blood Sugar Response: Monitor your blood sugar levels before and after meals to understand how different foods affect your body. Keep a food diary to track your intake and identify patterns or triggers that may impact your blood sugar control.

11. Individualized Approach: Work with a registered dietitian or healthcare provider to develop a personalized meal plan tailored to your nutritional

needs, lifestyle, cultural preferences, and diabetes management goals.

12. Regular Physical Activity: Combine healthy eating habits with regular physical activity to improve insulin sensitivity, manage weight, and enhance overall health and well-being.

By adopting a balanced and individualized approach to diet and nutrition, you can effectively manage your diabetes, optimize blood sugar control, and reduce the risk of complications while enjoying a varied and satisfying diet.

- Building a Diabetes-Friendly Diet

Building a diabetes-friendly diet involves choosing foods that help manage blood sugar levels, promote overall health, and reduce the risk of complications associated with diabetes. Here's how to create a balanced and nutritious meal plan:

1. Focus on Whole Foods: Base your diet around whole, minimally processed foods that are rich in nutrients and fiber.Make sure your meals contain an abundance of fruits, vegetables, whole grains, legumes, nuts, and seeds.

2. Choose Complex Carbohydrates: Opt for complex carbohydrates with a low glycemic index (GI), which are digested more slowly and cause gradual increases in blood sugar levels. Examples include whole grains (brown rice, quinoa, barley), legumes (beans, lentils), fruits, and vegetables.

3. Control Portion Sizes: Pay attention to portion sizes, especially when it comes to carbohydrate-containing foods, which have the most significant impact on blood sugar levels. Use measuring cups, food scales, or visual cues to help control portions and avoid overeating.

4. Include Lean Proteins: Incorporate lean protein sources into your meals to help stabilize blood sugar levels and promote satiety. Good options include poultry

(skinless chicken or turkey), fish, seafood, tofu, tempeh, beans, lentils, and low-fat dairy products.

5. Healthy Fats: Include sources of healthy fats in your diet, such as avocados, nuts, seeds, olive oil, and fatty fish like salmon and mackerel. Healthy fats support heart health and help improve insulin sensitivity.

6. Limit Saturated and Trans Fats: Minimize your intake of foods high in saturated and trans fats, such as fatty meats, full-fat dairy products, processed foods, and fried foods. These fats have the potential to boost cholesterol and heart disease risk.

7. Watch Sodium Intake: Limit your consumption of high-sodium foods, as excess sodium can contribute to high blood pressure and increase the risk of heart disease. Choose fresh or minimally processed foods and use herbs, spices, and citrus juices to flavor dishes instead of salt.

8. Stay Hydrated: Drink plenty of water throughout the day to stay hydrated and support overall health. Limit

sugary drinks, sodas, and fruit juices, which can cause spikes in blood sugar levels.

9. Mindful Eating: Practice mindful eating by paying attention to hunger and fullness cues, eating slowly, and savoring each bite. This can encourage improved blood sugar regulation and help avoid overindulging.

10. Regular Meal Timing: Aim to eat meals and snacks at regular intervals throughout the day to maintain consistent blood sugar levels and prevent spikes or drops. Space meals evenly and avoid prolonged periods of fasting.

11. Limit Added Sugars: Minimize your intake of foods and beverages high in added sugars, such as sweets, desserts, sugary cereals, and sugary drinks. Opt for naturally sweet foods like fruits and limit added sugars to help control blood sugar levels.

12. Individualize Your Plan: Work with a registered dietitian or healthcare provider to develop a personalized meal plan tailored to your nutritional

needs, lifestyle, cultural preferences, and diabetes management goals.

By incorporating these principles into your daily eating habits, you can create a diabetes-friendly diet that supports optimal blood sugar control, promotes overall health, and enhances your quality of life.

- Importance of Carbohydrate Counting

Carbohydrate counting is a valuable tool for individuals with diabetes to manage blood sugar levels effectively. Here's why it's important:

1. Impact on Blood Sugar: Carbohydrates are the main nutrient that affects blood sugar levels. Carbohydrates are converted in the body into glucose, which enters the bloodstream and elevates blood sugar. By counting carbohydrates, individuals can better predict and control their blood sugar response to meals and snacks.

2. Precision in Insulin Dosing: For individuals using insulin therapy, carbohydrate counting allows for more

precise dosing of insulin based on the amount of carbohydrates consumed. Matching insulin doses to carbohydrate intake helps prevent blood sugar spikes after meals and promotes better blood sugar control throughout the day.

3. Flexibility in Meal Planning: Carbohydrate counting provides flexibility in meal planning by allowing individuals to enjoy a variety of foods while still managing blood sugar levels effectively. Rather than focusing on specific foods to avoid, such as sugar or starches, individuals can focus on portion sizes and carbohydrate content within their overall meal plan.

4. Individualized Approach: Carbohydrate needs vary from person to person based on factors such as age, weight, activity level, medication regimen, and insulin sensitivity. Carbohydrate counting allows for a personalized approach to diabetes management, where individuals can adjust their carbohydrate intake to meet their unique needs and preferences.

5. Empowerment and Control: By learning how to count carbohydrates and understand their impact on blood sugar levels, individuals with diabetes gain a sense of empowerment and control over their condition. They become active participants in their diabetes management, making informed decisions about food choices, portion sizes, and insulin dosing.

6. Integration with Technology: Advances in technology, such as carbohydrate counting apps, food databases, and insulin pumps with bolus calculators, make it easier for individuals to track carbohydrates and calculate insulin doses accurately. These tools can streamline the carbohydrate counting process and enhance diabetes self-management.

7. Improved Glycemic Control: Studies have shown that carbohydrate counting, when combined with insulin therapy or other diabetes medications, can lead to improved glycemic control, lower HbA1c levels, and reduced risk of diabetes complications. Consistent carbohydrate counting helps stabilize blood sugar levels and minimize fluctuations throughout the day.

Overall, carbohydrate counting is a valuable skill for individuals with diabetes to learn and incorporate into their daily routine. It provides a practical and flexible approach to managing blood sugar levels, supporting overall health and well-being in the management of diabetes.

- Superfoods for Diabetics

While there's no single "superfood" that can cure diabetes, certain nutrient-rich foods can be particularly beneficial for managing blood sugar levels and promoting overall health in individuals with diabetes. Here are some examples:

1. Non-Starchy Vegetables: Non-starchy vegetables are low in carbohydrates and calories but high in fiber, vitamins, and minerals. They have minimal impact on blood sugar levels and can help promote satiety. Examples include leafy greens (spinach, kale, lettuce), broccoli, cauliflower, bell peppers, cucumbers, and tomatoes.

2. Berries: Berries are rich in antioxidants, fiber, and vitamins, making them an excellent choice for individuals with diabetes. Compared to other fruits, they have a lower glycemic index, which means their effect on blood sugar levels is less pronounced. Examples include strawberries, blueberries, raspberries, and blackberries.

3. Whole Grains: Whole grains are a good source of complex carbohydrates, fiber, and nutrients. They're digested more slowly than refined grains, leading to gradual increases in blood sugar levels. Choose whole grains such as oats, barley, quinoa, brown rice, whole wheat bread, and whole grain pasta.

4. Legumes: Legumes, including beans, lentils, and chickpeas, are high in fiber, protein, and complex carbohydrates. They can aid in blood sugar stabilization because they have a low glycemic index. Incorporate legumes into soups, stews, salads, and side dishes for added nutrition and satiety.

5. Fatty Fish: Fatty fish like salmon, mackerel, sardines, and trout are rich in omega-3 fatty acids, which have anti-inflammatory properties and may help reduce the risk of heart disease in individuals with diabetes. Try to eat seafood that is high in fat twice a week or more.

6. Nuts and Seeds: Nuts and seeds are packed with healthy fats, protein, fiber, and essential nutrients. They can help improve insulin sensitivity, promote heart health, and aid in weight management. Examples include almonds, walnuts, chia seeds, flaxseeds, and pumpkin seeds.

7. Greek Yogurt: Greek yogurt is high in protein and low in carbohydrates, making it a nutritious option for individuals with diabetes. Choose plain, unsweetened Greek yogurt and add fresh fruit, nuts, or seeds for natural sweetness and extra flavor.

8. Cinnamon: Cinnamon has been shown to improve insulin sensitivity and lower blood sugar levels in individuals with diabetes. Sprinkle cinnamon on

oatmeal, yogurt, or smoothies for added flavor and potential health benefits.

9. Green Tea: Green tea contains antioxidants called catechins, which may help improve insulin sensitivity and reduce the risk of cardiovascular disease in individuals with diabetes. Drink green tea as a refreshing beverage or add it to smoothies for a boost of antioxidants.

10. Avocado: Avocado is rich in heart-healthy monounsaturated fats, fiber, and potassium. It can help improve lipid profiles, lower cholesterol levels, and promote satiety. Scoop avocados for toast, include them in salads, or puree them into smoothies.

Incorporating these nutrient-rich foods into your diet as part of a well-balanced meal plan can help support blood sugar control, reduce the risk of complications associated with diabetes, and promote overall health and well-being. It's important to work with a registered dietitian or healthcare provider to develop a personalized meal plan that meets your individual nutritional needs, lifestyle, and diabetes management goals.

2.4 Exercise and Physical Activity

Exercise and physical activity are essential components of diabetes management, offering numerous benefits for both physical and mental health. Here's why exercise is important for individuals with diabetes:

1. Improved Blood Sugar Control: Exercise helps lower blood sugar levels by increasing insulin sensitivity, allowing glucose to be taken up by muscles for energy. Regular physical activity can lead to more stable blood sugar levels, reducing the risk of hyperglycemia (high blood sugar) and hypoglycemia (low blood sugar) episodes.

2. Weight Management: Exercise plays a key role in weight management by burning calories and promoting fat loss. Maintaining a healthy weight can improve insulin sensitivity, reduce insulin resistance, and lower

the risk of obesity-related complications such as heart disease and stroke.

3. Enhanced Cardiovascular Health: Regular exercise can improve cardiovascular health by strengthening the heart, lowering blood pressure, and improving circulation. It reduces the risk of cardiovascular disease, which is more prevalent in individuals with diabetes.

4. Improved Lipid Profile: Exercise can help raise HDL (good) cholesterol levels and lower LDL (bad) cholesterol levels, reducing the risk of atherosclerosis (hardening of the arteries) and cardiovascular disease.

5. Increased Muscle Strength and Endurance: Strength training exercises, such as weightlifting or resistance training, can help increase muscle mass, strength, and endurance. This not only improves overall physical function but also enhances metabolic health by increasing resting metabolic rate and insulin sensitivity.

6. Stress Reduction: Exercise has been shown to reduce stress, anxiety, and depression, all of which are common

among individuals with diabetes. Endorphins are neurotransmitters that are released in response to physical activity and are known to enhance emotions of happiness and wellbeing.

7. Improved Sleep Quality: Regular exercise can help improve sleep quality and duration, which is important for overall health and blood sugar control. Adequate sleep supports hormone regulation, including insulin production and sensitivity.

8. Enhanced Diabetes Management: Exercise complements other aspects of diabetes management, including medication or insulin therapy, meal planning, and blood sugar monitoring. When combined with a healthy diet and medication regimen, regular physical activity can help individuals achieve better overall diabetes control.

9. Reduced Risk of Complications: By improving blood sugar control, cardiovascular health, weight management, and overall well-being, exercise can help reduce the risk of diabetes-related complications such as

heart disease, stroke, nerve damage, kidney disease, and vision problems.

10. Increased Longevity and Quality of Life: Regular exercise has been associated with a longer lifespan and improved quality of life in individuals with diabetes. It promotes independence, mobility, and vitality, allowing individuals to better manage their condition and enjoy an active lifestyle.

It's important for individuals with diabetes to engage in regular physical activity as part of their overall diabetes management plan. Before starting an exercise program, consult with a healthcare provider to ensure it's safe and appropriate for your individual health status and fitness level. Aim for a combination of aerobic exercise, strength training, flexibility, and balance exercises to reap the full benefits of physical activity.

- Benefits of Exercise

Exercise offers numerous benefits for both physical and mental health, regardless of whether you have diabetes.

The following are some main advantages of consistent exercise:

1. Improved Cardiovascular Health: Exercise strengthens the heart muscle, improves circulation, and lowers blood pressure, reducing the risk of heart disease, heart attack, and stroke.

2. Better Blood Sugar Control: Physical activity helps lower blood sugar levels by increasing insulin sensitivity and glucose uptake by muscles, reducing the risk of hyperglycemia (high blood sugar) and improving overall diabetes management.

3. Weight Management: Exercise burns calories, promotes fat loss, and increases muscle mass, helping to achieve and maintain a healthy weight. It also boosts metabolism, making it easier to manage weight over the long term.

4. Increased Muscle Strength and Endurance: Strength training exercises build muscle mass, strength, and

endurance, enhancing physical performance, mobility, and functional capacity.

5. Improved Bone Health: Weight-bearing exercises, such as walking, jogging, and strength training, help build and maintain bone density, reducing the risk of osteoporosis and fractures.

6. Enhanced Mental Health: Exercise stimulates the release of endorphins, neurotransmitters that promote feelings of well-being and happiness. It reduces stress, anxiety, and depression, improving mood and mental resilience.

7. Better Sleep Quality: Regular exercise can improve sleep quality and duration, leading to more restful and refreshing sleep. It helps regulate circadian rhythms and promotes relaxation, making it easier to fall asleep and stay asleep.

8. Increased Energy Levels: Exercise increases energy levels by improving circulation, oxygen delivery, and nutrient uptake throughout the body. It boosts stamina,

endurance, and vitality, reducing fatigue and enhancing overall productivity and performance.

9. Enhanced Immune Function: Moderate-intensity exercise strengthens the immune system, reducing the risk of infections and illnesses. It promotes the production of white blood cells and antibodies, enhancing the body's ability to fight off pathogens.

10. Reduced Risk of Chronic Diseases: Regular exercise lowers the risk of chronic diseases such as type 2 diabetes, obesity, hypertension, dyslipidemia, and certain types of cancer. It improves overall health and longevity, extending lifespan and reducing healthcare costs.

11. Social Connection: Exercise provides opportunities for social interaction and community engagement, whether through group fitness classes, sports teams, or outdoor activities. It fosters friendships, teamwork, and a sense of belonging, contributing to overall well-being and quality of life.

12. Increased Longevity: Regular physical activity has been associated with a longer lifespan and improved quality of life in both younger and older adults. It promotes healthy aging, independence, and vitality, allowing individuals to enjoy a full and active life.

Incorporating regular exercise into your routine can have profound benefits for your physical and mental health, regardless of age, fitness level, or medical condition. Aim for a combination of aerobic exercise, strength training, flexibility, and balance exercises to reap the full spectrum of benefits and enjoy a healthier, happier life.

- **Types of Suitable Exercises**

There are various types of exercises suitable for individuals with diabetes, each offering unique benefits for overall health and blood sugar control. Here are some examples of suitable exercises for people with diabetes:

1. Aerobic Exercise:

- Walking: Easily incorporated into daily life, walking is a low-impact exercise. On most days of the week, try to get in at least 30 minutes of vigorous walking.
- Cycling: Cycling is a great cardiovascular exercise that can be done indoors on a stationary bike or outdoors on a bicycle.
- Swimming: Swimming is a low-impact, full-body exercise that benefits joints. It's particularly beneficial for individuals with arthritis or mobility issues.
- Dancing: Dancing is a fun and social way to get your heart pumping and burn calories. Choose dance styles like Zumba, salsa, or ballroom dancing.
- Elliptical Training: Elliptical machines provide a low-impact cardiovascular workout that engages both the upper and lower body muscles.

2. Strength Training:
- Bodyweight Exercises: Exercises like squats, lunges, push-ups, and planks can be done using your body weight for resistance.
- Resistance Bands: Resistance bands provide resistance during strength training exercises and are portable and versatile.

- Free Weights: Dumbbells, kettlebells, and barbells can be used to perform a variety of strength training exercises targeting different muscle groups.

- Weight Machines: Strength training machines at the gym offer guided resistance exercises for various muscle groups.

3. Flexibility and Stretching:

- Yoga: Yoga improves flexibility, balance, and strength while promoting relaxation and stress reduction.
- Pilates: Using deliberate movements and breathing exercises, Pilates emphasizes body awareness, flexibility, and core strength.
- Tai Chi: Tai Chi is a gentle exercise that combines deep breathing and slow, flowing motions. It improves balance, flexibility, and mental focus.

4. Balance Exercises:

- Balance Exercises: Standing on one leg, heel-to-toe walking, and using balance boards or stability balls can help improve balance and reduce the risk of falls.

- Tai Chi: Tai Chi exercises are also beneficial for improving balance and coordination.

5. Interval Training:
  - High-Intensity Interval Training (HIIT): HIIT involves alternating short bursts of intense exercise with periods of rest or lower-intensity exercise. It can be performed with a variety of exercises, such as bodyweight movements, cycling, or running.
  - Tabata: Tabata training is a specific form of HIIT that consists of 20 seconds of intense exercise followed by 10 seconds of rest, repeated for multiple rounds.

6. Sports and Recreational Activities:
  - Tennis: Tennis is a dynamic sport that provides cardiovascular exercise, strength training, and agility.
  - Golf: Golfing involves walking, swinging, and carrying or pulling clubs, providing moderate physical activity.
  - Team Sports: Team sports like soccer, basketball, and volleyball offer aerobic exercise, strength training, and social interaction.

When starting an exercise program, it's essential to consult with a healthcare provider, especially if you have any existing health conditions or concerns. They can help you choose appropriate exercises, set realistic goals, and ensure your safety during physical activity. Aim for a combination of aerobic, strength, flexibility, and balance exercises to enjoy a well-rounded fitness routine that supports your overall health and diabetes management goals.

- Creating a Workout Plan

Creating a workout plan involves setting specific goals, selecting suitable exercises, scheduling workouts, and gradually increasing intensity over time. Here's a step-by-step guide to creating a personalized workout plan:

1. Set Goals:
   - Determine what you want to achieve with your workout plan. Your goals could include improving cardiovascular health, building strength, increasing flexibility, managing weight, or enhancing overall fitness.

- Make your goals specific, measurable, achievable, relevant, and time-bound (SMART) to help guide your progress and keep you motivated.

2. Assess Your Current Fitness Level:
   - Evaluate your current fitness level, including your cardiovascular endurance, strength, flexibility, and balance.
   - Consider any health concerns, medical conditions, or physical limitations that may impact your ability to exercise. Consult with a healthcare provider if you have any concerns or need guidance.

3. Choose Suitable Exercises:
   - Select exercises that align with your goals and preferences. Include a variety of cardiovascular, strength training, flexibility, and balance exercises to create a well-rounded workout plan.
   - Consider your fitness level, interests, equipment availability, and any physical limitations when choosing exercises.
   - Aim for a mix of aerobic activities (e.g., walking, cycling, swimming), strength training exercises (e.g.,

bodyweight exercises, resistance training), flexibility exercises (e.g., yoga, stretching), and balance exercises (e.g., Tai Chi, stability exercises).

4. Plan Your Workouts:
   - Determine how many days per week you'll exercise and how long each workout session will be. Aim for at least 150 minutes of moderate-intensity aerobic exercise or 75 minutes of vigorous-intensity aerobic exercise per week, along with strength training exercises on two or more days per week.
   - Schedule your workouts at times that fit into your daily routine and allow for consistency. Consider morning, afternoon, or evening workouts based on your energy levels and schedule.
   - Vary your exercise routines to avoid monotony and maintain interest. Alternate between different types of exercise, intensity levels, and workout formats (e.g., circuit training, interval training, group classes).

5. Gradually Increase Intensity:
   - Start with manageable levels of intensity, duration, and frequency, especially if you're new to exercise or

returning after a break. Gradually increase the intensity and duration of your workouts over time as your fitness level improves.

   - Use the principle of progressive overload to challenge your body and stimulate adaptation. Increase the intensity, duration, or resistance of your workouts gradually to continue making progress.

6. Include Rest and Recovery:
   - Schedule rest days and recovery periods into your workout plan to allow your body time to repair and rebuild muscle tissue, replenish energy stores, and prevent overtraining.
   - Listen to your body and adjust your workout intensity or schedule as needed based on how you feel. Pay attention to signs of fatigue, soreness, or injury, and give yourself permission to take rest days when necessary.

7. Track Your Progress:
 Maintain a log of your exercises, advancements, and successes to keep yourself accountable and inspired. Use a workout journal, fitness app, or wearable fitness

tracker to record your workouts, track your performance, and monitor changes over time.

- Celebrate your successes and milestones along the way, whether it's reaching a fitness goal, increasing the weight lifted, or improving your endurance.

8. Modify and Adapt:

- Be flexible and willing to adjust your workout plan as needed based on your changing goals, preferences, and circumstances. Modify exercises, intensity levels, or workout formats to keep your routine fresh and challenging.

- Consult with a fitness professional or personal trainer for guidance and support in developing and modifying your workout plan as needed.

By following these steps, you can create a personalized workout plan that aligns with your goals, fits into your lifestyle, and supports your overall health and well-being. Remember to listen to your body, stay consistent, and enjoy the journey of improving your fitness and reaching your goals.

Chapter 3:

Living Well with Diabetes

Living well with diabetes involves adopting a holistic approach to managing the condition and prioritizing overall health and well-being. Here are some key strategies for effectively managing diabetes and optimizing your quality of life:

1. Education and Awareness:
   - Learn as much as you can about diabetes, including its causes, symptoms, treatment options, and potential complications. Understanding the condition empowers you to make informed decisions about your health and effectively manage your diabetes.

2. Blood Sugar Monitoring:
   - Monitor your blood sugar levels regularly as recommended by your healthcare provider. Keeping track of your blood sugar levels helps you understand

how food, physical activity, medications, and other factors affect your diabetes management.

3. Healthy Eating Habits:
   - Follow a balanced and nutritious diet that emphasizes whole foods, including fruits, vegetables, whole grains, lean proteins, and healthy fats. Limit your intake of refined carbohydrates, sugars, saturated fats, and processed foods. Consider working with a registered dietitian to develop a personalized meal plan that meets your nutritional needs and diabetes management goals.

4. Regular Physical Activity:
   - Engage in regular physical activity to help control blood sugar levels, improve insulin sensitivity, manage weight, and enhance overall health. Aim for at least 150 minutes of moderate-intensity aerobic exercise or 75 minutes of vigorous-intensity exercise per week, as recommended by guidelines. Incorporate activities you enjoy, such as walking, cycling, swimming, or dancing, into your routine.

5. Weight Management:

  -If you are overweight or obese, try to maintain a healthy weight or strive towards reaching one. Losing even a modest amount of weight can improve insulin sensitivity, reduce blood sugar levels, and lower the risk of diabetes-related complications. Make sustainable lifestyle choices, including eating a more balanced diet and exercising more, your main priority.

6. Medication Adherence:

  - Take your diabetes medications as prescribed by your healthcare provider and follow their instructions carefully. Oral medications, insulin therapy, and other medications help control blood sugar levels and prevent complications. Discuss any worries you may have or any adverse effects you may be experiencing with your healthcare provider.

7. Stress Management:

  - Practice stress-reducing techniques such as deep breathing, meditation, yoga, mindfulness, or progressive muscle relaxation to manage stress effectively. Chronic stress can raise blood sugar levels and interfere with diabetes management, so it's essential to find healthy ways to cope with stress.

8. Regular Healthcare Checkups:
   - Attend regular checkups with your healthcare provider to monitor your diabetes management, assess your overall health, and screen for diabetes-related complications. Discuss any concerns or questions you may have about your diabetes management during these appointments.

9. Support Network:
   - Create a solid support system consisting of friends, family, medical professionals, and diabetic support organizations. Surrounding yourself with supportive individuals who understand your challenges and can provide encouragement, guidance, and assistance can make a significant difference in managing diabetes.

10. Positive Outlook and Self-Care:
   - Maintain a positive outlook and practice self-care to nurture your physical, emotional, and mental well-being. Make time for activities you enjoy, prioritize relaxation

and leisure, get adequate sleep, and seek professional help if you're struggling with diabetes-related stress, anxiety, or depression.

By incorporating these strategies into your daily life, you can effectively manage your diabetes, reduce the risk of complications, and live a fulfilling life. Remember that diabetes management is a journey, and it's essential to be patient, persistent, and proactive in caring for your health.

3.1 Creating a Diabetes Management Plan

Creating a personalized diabetes management plan involves collaborating with your healthcare team to develop strategies that address your individual needs, preferences, and health goals. Here's a step-by-step guide to help you create a comprehensive diabetes management plan:

1. Establish Goals:

- Begin by defining clear and achievable goals for managing your diabetes. These goals may include achieving target blood sugar levels, maintaining a healthy weight, improving lifestyle habits (such as diet and exercise), reducing the risk of complications, and enhancing overall well-being.

2. Work with Your Healthcare Team:
   - Consult with your healthcare provider, diabetes educator, registered dietitian, and other members of your healthcare team to develop your management plan. They can provide valuable guidance, support, and expertise to help you navigate the complexities of diabetes management.

3. Blood Sugar Monitoring:
   - Determine how often you will monitor your blood sugar levels based on your healthcare provider's recommendations and your individual needs. Use a blood glucose meter to measure your blood sugar levels at home and keep a record of your results to track patterns over time.

4. Medication Management:

   - Discuss your medication regimen with your healthcare provider and ensure that you understand how to take your medications correctly. Oral medicine, insulin therapy, and other injectable drugs may fall under this category. Follow your provider's instructions for dosing, timing, and potential side effects.

5. Meal Planning:

   - Develop a balanced meal plan that aligns with your nutritional needs, blood sugar targets, and personal preferences. Aim to eat a variety of nutrient-rich foods, including fruits, vegetables, whole grains, lean proteins, and healthy fats. Consider working with a registered dietitian to create a customized meal plan that fits your lifestyle and diabetes management goals.

6. Physical Activity:

   - Incorporate regular physical activity into your routine to help control blood sugar levels, manage weight, and improve overall health. Choose activities you enjoy and aim for a combination of aerobic exercise, strength training, and flexibility exercises. Set realistic goals and gradually increase your activity level over time.

7. Stress Management:
   - Implement stress-reducing techniques such as deep breathing, meditation, yoga, or mindfulness to manage stress effectively. Chronic stress can affect blood sugar levels and interfere with diabetes management, so it's essential to find healthy ways to cope with stress.

8. Regular Healthcare Checkups:
   - Schedule regular checkups with your healthcare provider to monitor your diabetes management, assess your overall health, and screen for diabetes-related complications. Discuss any concerns or questions you may have about your diabetes management during these appointments.

9. Emergency Preparedness:
   - Develop a plan for managing diabetes-related emergencies, such as hypoglycemia (low blood sugar) or hyperglycemia (high blood sugar). Carry medical identification, such as a diabetes alert bracelet or

necklace, and keep emergency contact information readily available.

10. Ongoing Education and Support:
   - Stay informed about diabetes management through ongoing education, support groups, and resources provided by your healthcare team, reputable organizations (such as the American Diabetes Association), and online communities. Seek support from family, friends, and peers who understand your journey and can provide encouragement and guidance.

By following these steps and actively engaging in your diabetes management, you can develop a comprehensive plan that empowers you to take control of your health and live well with diabetes. Remember that diabetes management is a continuous process, and it's essential to adapt your plan as needed based on changes in your health, lifestyle, and treatment goals.

- **Setting Realistic Goals**

Setting realistic goals is crucial for successful diabetes management, as it helps you stay motivated, track progress, and achieve meaningful outcomes. Here's how to set realistic goals for managing diabetes:

1. Be Specific:
  - Clearly and precisely state your objectives. Instead of a vague goal like "improve blood sugar control," specify what you want to achieve, such as "lower fasting blood sugar levels to below 120 mg/dL."

2. Make Them Measurable:
  Make sure your objectives are quantifiable so you can monitor your development over time. Use quantifiable metrics such as blood sugar levels, weight, exercise duration, or servings of fruits and vegetables.

3. Set Achievable Goals:
  - Be realistic about what you can accomplish given your current circumstances, resources, and limitations. Set goals that are challenging yet attainable, considering factors such as your health status, lifestyle, and available support.

4. Break Them Down:

   - Break larger goals into smaller, manageable steps or milestones. This lessens their overpowering nature and enables you to acknowledge your accomplishments as you go. For example, if your long-term goal is to lose 20 pounds, set smaller monthly weight loss targets.

5. Prioritize:

   Decide which objectives are most important to you, then give those your whole attention. Prioritize goals based on their impact on your health, quality of life, and overall well-being. Addressing the most critical goals can help you build momentum and confidence.

6. Be Flexible:

   - Remain flexible and adaptable in your goal-setting process. Recognize that progress may not always follow a linear path, and setbacks or obstacles may arise. Adjust your goals as needed based on changes in your health, circumstances, or treatment plan.

7. Set Timeframes:

- Establish realistic timelines for achieving your goals. Consider short-term, medium-term, and long-term timeframes based on the complexity of the goal and your ability to work towards it consistently.

8. Celebrate Successes:
   - No matter how tiny, recognize and celebrate your accomplishments. Recognizing progress and celebrating milestones can boost your motivation and reinforce positive behaviors. Reward yourself for reaching your goals with non-food rewards or activities you enjoy.

9. Stay Positive:
   - Maintain a positive attitude and mindset throughout your diabetes management journey. Focus on what you can control and celebrate your efforts, even if you encounter setbacks or challenges along the way. Stay resilient and keep moving forward.

10. Seek Support:
   - Don't hesitate to seek support from your healthcare team, family, friends, or peers. Share your goals with others who can provide encouragement, accountability,

and practical assistance. Having a supportive network can make a significant difference in achieving your goals.

By setting realistic and achievable goals, you can effectively manage your diabetes, improve your health outcomes, and enhance your overall well-being. Remember that progress takes time, patience, and perseverance, so be kind to yourself and celebrate every step forward on your journey towards better health.

- Keeping Track of Your Progress

Keeping track of your progress is essential for monitoring your diabetes management efforts, identifying trends, and making informed adjustments to your treatment plan. The following are some practical methods for monitoring your development:

1. Blood Sugar Monitoring:
   - As directed by your physician, check your blood sugar levels on a regular basis. Use a blood glucose meter to measure your fasting blood sugar levels, pre-

meal levels, post-meal levels, and bedtime levels. Record your readings in a blood sugar log or mobile app to track patterns over time.

2. Food Diary:

   - Keep a food diary to track your dietary intake and monitor how different foods affect your blood sugar levels. Record what you eat, portion sizes, carbohydrate counts, and meal timings. Use a paper journal, smartphone app, or online tool to log your meals and snacks.

3. Physical Activity Log:

   - Maintain a physical activity log to track your exercise habits and monitor your activity levels. Record the type of exercise, duration, intensity, and frequency of your workouts. Include activities such as walking, cycling, swimming, strength training, and flexibility exercises.

4. Medication and Insulin Records:

   - Keep a record of your medication and insulin doses, including the type, dosage, frequency, and timing of administration. Note any changes in your medication regimen, as well as any side effects or adverse reactions you experience.

5. Weight and Measurements:

- Track your weight, body measurements, and body mass index (BMI) regularly to monitor changes in your body composition. Use a scale, measuring tape, or body composition analyzer to record your weight, waist circumference, hip circumference, and other relevant measurements.

6. Symptom Tracker:

- Keep a symptom tracker to monitor any diabetes-related symptoms or complications you experience. Note the type and severity of symptoms, as well as any triggers or patterns you observe. This can help you identify early warning signs and alert your healthcare provider to potential issues.

7. A1c Test Results:

- Schedule regular A1c tests (glycated hemoglobin tests) to assess your average blood sugar levels over the past two to three months. Keep track of your A1c results and discuss them with your healthcare provider to evaluate your diabetes management and adjust your treatment plan if necessary.

8. Mood and Well-being:
   - Pay attention to your mood, emotions, and overall well-being as they relate to your diabetes management. Keep a journal to track your feelings, stress levels, energy levels, and quality of life. Consider seeking support from a therapist or counselor if you're struggling with diabetes-related emotional challenges.

9. Goals and Progress Notes:
   - Document your diabetes management goals, progress, and achievements in a goals journal or progress tracker. Review your goals regularly and update them as needed based on changes in your health, lifestyle, or treatment plan.

10. Regular Check-ins with Healthcare Team:
   - Schedule regular check-ins with your healthcare provider and other members of your healthcare team to review your progress, discuss any concerns or

challenges, and make adjustments to your diabetes management plan. Share your progress logs and records with your healthcare team during these appointments.

By keeping track of your progress using these strategies, you can gain valuable insights into your diabetes management efforts, identify areas for improvement, and work towards achieving your health goals. Remember that consistency, patience, and persistence are key to successful diabetes management, so continue to monitor your progress and make adjustments as needed to optimize your health and well-being.

3.2 Coping with the Emotional Impact

Coping with the emotional impact of diabetes is an important aspect of overall diabetes management. Living with a chronic condition like diabetes can bring about various emotional challenges, including stress, anxiety, depression, frustration, fear, and feelings of isolation. Here are some strategies to help cope with the emotional impact of diabetes:

1. Education and Understanding:
   - Educate yourself about diabetes to gain a better understanding of the condition, its management, and its impact on your life. Knowledge empowers you to make informed decisions, feel more in control, and reduce anxiety about the unknown.

2. Seek Support:
   - Reach out to family, friends, and peers who can provide emotional support, encouragement, and understanding. Joining a diabetes support group or online community can also connect you with others who are facing similar challenges and provide a sense of belonging.

3. Communicate Openly:
   - Share your feelings, concerns, and experiences with trusted individuals, including your healthcare team, family members, and friends. Open communication

allows others to offer support, validate your emotions, and provide practical assistance when needed.

4. Practice Stress Management Techniques:
   - To effectively manage stress, incorporate ways for minimizing it into your everyday routine. This may include deep breathing exercises, meditation, mindfulness, progressive muscle relaxation, yoga, or tai chi. Find activities that help you relax and unwind, and prioritize self-care.

5. Focus on the Positive:
   - Cultivate a positive mindset and focus on the aspects of your life that bring joy, fulfillment, and gratitude. Celebrate your achievements, no matter how small, and acknowledge your strengths and resilience in managing diabetes.

6. Set Realistic Expectations:
   - Set realistic expectations for yourself and your diabetes management. Understand that managing diabetes is a journey with ups and downs, and it's okay

to have setbacks or challenges along the way. Take it one step at a time and practice self-compassion.

7. Engage in Activities You Enjoy:
   - Make time for activities and hobbies that bring you pleasure, relaxation, and a sense of purpose. Engaging in enjoyable activities can help distract from diabetes-related stressors and boost your mood and well-being.

8. Practice Self-Compassion:
   - Be kind to yourself and practice self-compassion in your diabetes journey. Recognize that living with diabetes can be challenging at times, and it's okay to experience a range of emotions. Be nice and understanding to yourself as you would a friend going through a similar ordeal.

9. Seek Professional Help if Needed:
   - If you're struggling to cope with the emotional impact of diabetes, consider seeking support from a mental health professional, such as a therapist or counselor. Therapy can provide a safe space to explore

your feelings, develop coping strategies, and work through challenges related to diabetes.

10. Stay Connected:
  - Stay connected with your healthcare team and attend regular check-ups to monitor your diabetes management and address any concerns or issues. Your healthcare team can offer guidance, support, and resources to help you cope with the emotional aspects of diabetes.

Remember that it's normal to experience a range of emotions when living with diabetes, and you're not alone in facing these challenges. By implementing these coping strategies and seeking support when needed, you can navigate the emotional impact of diabetes more effectively and improve your overall well-being.

- Managing Stress and Anxiety

Managing stress and anxiety is essential for overall well-being, especially when living with a chronic condition like diabetes. Here are some strategies to help manage stress and anxiety effectively:

1. Practice Relaxation Techniques:
  - To help you cope with stress and anxiety, incorporate relaxation techniques into your everyday routine. Deep breathing exercises, progressive muscle relaxation, guided imagery, and meditation are effective techniques for promoting relaxation and calmness.

2. Stay Active:
  - Engage in regular physical activity to help reduce stress and anxiety levels. Exercise encourages relaxation and releases endorphins, which are naturally occurring mood enhancers. Choose activities you enjoy, such as walking, jogging, yoga, swimming, or dancing, and aim for at least 30 minutes of moderate-intensity exercise most days of the week.

3. Maintain a Healthy Lifestyle:
  - Eat a balanced diet, get adequate sleep, and avoid excessive caffeine, alcohol, and nicotine, as they can contribute to stress and anxiety. Prioritize self-care

activities such as getting enough rest, eating nutritious meals, staying hydrated, and practicing good sleep hygiene.

4. Set Realistic Expectations:
   - Set realistic expectations for yourself and your diabetes management. Avoid perfectionism and accept that you may not always be able to control every aspect of your diabetes. Prioritize progress above perfection and acknowledge and appreciate all of your accomplishments, no matter how tiny.

5. Practice Mindfulness:
   - Practice mindfulness techniques to help stay present and grounded in the moment. Mindfulness involves paying attention to your thoughts, feelings, bodily sensations, and the environment without judgment. Mindfulness meditation, mindful eating, and body scans are effective practices for reducing stress and anxiety.

6. Seek Social Support:
   - Reach out to family, friends, and peers for emotional support and companionship. Talking to others about

your feelings and concerns can help alleviate stress and provide a sense of connection and understanding. Joining a diabetes support group or online community can also offer valuable support and encouragement.

7. Time Management:

   - Prioritize tasks and manage your time effectively to reduce feelings of overwhelm and stress. Break tasks into smaller, manageable steps, set realistic deadlines, and delegate tasks when possible. Use tools such as calendars, planners, or smartphone apps to organize your schedule and stay on track.

8. Limit Exposure to Stressors:

   Determine the sources of stress in your life and, if at all possible, take action to reduce or eliminate them. This may involve setting boundaries, saying no to excessive commitments, avoiding stressful situations or people, and making time for activities that bring you joy and relaxation.

9. Practice Assertiveness:

- Learn to assert yourself and communicate your needs, boundaries, and concerns effectively. Assertive communication can help reduce feelings of resentment, frustration, and anxiety in interpersonal relationships and promote healthier interactions with others.

10. Seek Professional Help if Needed:
   - If stress and anxiety persist or significantly impact your daily life, consider seeking support from a mental health professional, such as a therapist or counselor. Therapy can provide coping strategies, support, and guidance to help you manage stress and anxiety more effectively.

By incorporating these strategies into your daily life, you can better manage stress and anxiety, improve your overall well-being, and enhance your ability to cope with the challenges of living with diabetes. Remember that it's okay to ask for help when needed and prioritize self-care to support your mental and emotional health.

- Finding Support and Resources

Finding support and resources is crucial for managing diabetes effectively and coping with its emotional, physical, and practical challenges. Here are some strategies to help you find support and access valuable resources:

1. Healthcare Team:
   - Your healthcare team, including your primary care physician, endocrinologist, diabetes educator, registered dietitian, and other specialists, can provide valuable support, guidance, and resources to help you manage diabetes. Schedule regular appointments to discuss your diabetes management, ask questions, and address concerns.

2. Diabetes Education Programs:
   - Participate in diabetes education programs offered by healthcare facilities, community organizations, or online platforms. These programs provide information, resources, and support to help you understand diabetes, develop self-management skills, and make informed decisions about your health.

3. Support Groups:

   - Join a diabetes support group or online community to connect with others who are living with diabetes. These groups offer a supportive environment where you can share experiences, exchange tips and advice, and receive encouragement from peers who understand what you're going through.

4. National Organizations:

   - Explore resources and support services provided by national diabetes organizations such as the American Diabetes Association (ADA), the Juvenile Diabetes Research Foundation (JDRF), and the American Association of Diabetes Educators (AADE). These organizations offer educational materials, online forums, helplines, and local chapters that provide support and advocacy for individuals with diabetes.

5. Online Resources:

   - Take advantage of online resources and websites dedicated to diabetes education, management, and support. Websites such as Diabetes.org, Mayo Clinic, WebMD, and Diabetes.co.uk offer comprehensive information, articles, videos, tools, and community forums to help you navigate life with diabetes.

6. Mobile Apps:

   - Explore diabetes management apps and mobile tools that can help you track blood sugar levels, monitor food intake, log physical activity, and manage medications. Many apps also offer educational content, reminders, and personalized insights to support your diabetes management efforts.

7. Books and Publications:

   - Read books, magazines, and publications about diabetes written by experts, healthcare professionals, and individuals with lived experience. Look for titles that cover topics such as diabetes self-management, nutrition, exercise, mental health, and coping strategies.

8. Community Resources:

   - Investigate local community resources, such as diabetes clinics, support groups, wellness programs, and health fairs. Community organizations, churches, schools, and libraries may also offer diabetes-related workshops, classes, and events that provide valuable information and support.

9. Counseling and Therapy:
   - Consider seeking support from a mental health professional, such as a therapist or counselor, if you're struggling with the emotional impact of diabetes. Therapy can provide coping strategies, emotional support, and a safe space to explore your feelings and concerns related to diabetes.

10. Peer Support:
   - Connect with friends, family members, or colleagues who can offer practical assistance, encouragement, and empathy as you navigate life with diabetes. Share your experiences, communicate your needs, and lean on your support network when you need help or encouragement.

By accessing support and resources from various sources, you can enhance your diabetes management skills, improve your quality of life, and feel more empowered to navigate the challenges of living with diabetes. Remember that you're not alone, and there are many people and organizations available to help you along your diabetes journey.

3.3 Preventing Complications

Preventing complications is a critical aspect of managing diabetes effectively and maintaining long-term health and well-being. Here are some key strategies for preventing complications associated with diabetes:

1. Blood Sugar Control:
   - Maintain good blood sugar control by monitoring your blood sugar levels regularly, following your diabetes management plan, and adhering to medication and insulin regimens as prescribed by your healthcare provider. Aim for target blood sugar levels recommended by your healthcare team to reduce the risk of complications.

2. Healthy Eating Habits:
   - Follow a balanced and nutritious diet that emphasizes whole foods, including fruits, vegetables,

whole grains, lean proteins, and healthy fats. Limit your intake of refined carbohydrates, sugars, saturated fats, and processed foods. Work with a registered dietitian to develop a personalized meal plan that supports blood sugar control and overall health.

3. Regular Physical Activity:

   - Engage in regular physical activity to help control blood sugar levels, improve insulin sensitivity, manage weight, and reduce the risk of cardiovascular complications. Aim for at least 150 minutes of moderate-intensity aerobic exercise or 75 minutes of vigorous-intensity exercise per week, as recommended by guidelines.

4. Weight Management:

   - If you are overweight or obese, try to maintain a healthy weight or reach your goal. Losing excess weight can improve blood sugar control, reduce insulin resistance, lower blood pressure, and decrease the risk of diabetes-related complications. Focus on making sustainable lifestyle changes, such as adopting a healthy diet and increasing physical activity.

5. Blood Pressure Management:

Maintain your blood pressure within the range that your healthcare practitioner has prescribed. High blood pressure (hypertension) is a common complication of diabetes and can increase the risk of cardiovascular disease, kidney disease, and other complications. Monitor your blood pressure regularly and follow your healthcare provider's recommendations for management.

6. Cholesterol Management:

- Maintain healthy cholesterol levels by following a heart-healthy diet, exercising regularly, and taking medications if prescribed by your healthcare provider. High cholesterol levels can increase the risk of heart disease, stroke, and other vascular complications in people with diabetes.

7. Smoking Cessation:

- If you smoke, quit smoking to reduce the risk of cardiovascular disease, stroke, peripheral artery disease, and other complications associated with diabetes.

Smoking increases inflammation, damages blood vessels, and worsens insulin resistance, making it harder to control blood sugar levels.

8. Regular Healthcare Checkups:
  - Attend regular checkups with your healthcare provider to monitor your diabetes management, assess your overall health, and screen for diabetes-related complications. Regular screenings for eye disease (diabetic retinopathy), kidney disease (diabetic nephropathy), nerve damage (diabetic neuropathy), and foot problems (diabetic foot) are essential for early detection and intervention.

9. Foot Care:
  - Take care of your feet by inspecting them daily for cuts, sores, blisters, or other signs of infection. Keep your feet clean and dry, wear comfortable, well-fitting shoes, and avoid walking barefoot. Report any foot problems to your healthcare provider promptly to prevent complications such as foot ulcers or infections.

10. Diabetes Education and Self-Management:

- Participate in diabetes education programs and self-management initiatives to learn about diabetes, develop self-care skills, and empower yourself to make informed decisions about your health. Education and self-management support can help you understand the importance of preventive measures and take proactive steps to prevent complications.

By implementing these preventive strategies and working closely with your healthcare team, you can reduce the risk of complications associated with diabetes and maintain optimal health and well-being over the long term. Remember that prevention is key, and early intervention can make a significant difference in reducing the impact of diabetes-related complications on your life.

- Common Complications and How to Avoid Them

Managing diabetes effectively can help prevent or delay the onset of complications associated with the condition. Here are some common complications of diabetes and strategies to avoid them:

1. Cardiovascular Disease:

   - Complications: Diabetes increases the risk of heart disease, heart attack, stroke, and peripheral artery disease.

   - Prevention: Maintain good blood sugar control, manage blood pressure and cholesterol levels, follow a heart-healthy diet low in saturated fats and sodium, engage in regular physical activity, quit smoking, and attend regular check-ups with your healthcare provider.

2. Diabetic Retinopathy:

   - Complications: Diabetes can damage the blood vessels in the retina, leading to vision problems and even blindness.

   - Prevention: Control blood sugar levels, maintain healthy blood pressure and cholesterol levels, undergo regular eye exams, and promptly treat any eye problems or changes in vision.

3. Diabetic Neuropathy:

- Complications: Diabetes can cause nerve damage, leading to symptoms such as numbness, tingling, pain, and loss of sensation in the extremities.
- Prevention: Control blood sugar levels, maintain good foot care habits, inspect feet daily for signs of injury or infection, wear properly fitting shoes, and avoid walking barefoot.

4. Diabetic Nephropathy (Kidney Disease):
- Complications: Diabetes can damage the kidneys, leading to reduced kidney function and eventually kidney failure.
- Prevention: Control blood sugar levels, manage blood pressure, maintain a healthy diet low in sodium and protein, limit alcohol intake, avoid smoking, and undergo regular kidney function tests.

5. Diabetic Foot Complications:
- Complications: Diabetes can cause poor circulation and nerve damage in the feet, increasing the risk of foot ulcers, infections, and amputations.
- Prevention: Inspect feet daily for cuts, sores, blisters, or other signs of injury, keep feet clean and dry, wear

properly fitting shoes, avoid walking barefoot, trim toenails carefully, and seek prompt medical attention for any foot problems.

6. Hypoglycemia (Low Blood Sugar):
   - Complications: Diabetes medications, insulin therapy, and lifestyle factors can sometimes cause blood sugar levels to drop too low, leading to symptoms such as dizziness, sweating, confusion, and loss of consciousness.
   - Prevention: Monitor blood sugar levels regularly, follow a consistent meal plan, be aware of the signs and symptoms of hypoglycemia, carry fast-acting carbohydrates for emergencies, and adjust medication dosages as directed by your healthcare provider as needed.

7. Hyperglycemia (High Blood Sugar):
   - Complications: Prolonged high blood sugar levels can damage blood vessels and organs, leading to complications such as diabetic ketoacidosis (DKA) and hyperosmolar hyperglycemic state (HHS).

- Prevention: Monitor blood sugar levels regularly, adhere to your diabetes management plan, take medications as prescribed, follow a healthy diet, engage in regular physical activity, and seek medical attention if blood sugar levels remain consistently high.

8. Infections:
   - Complications: Diabetes can weaken the immune system, increasing the risk of infections, particularly in the skin, urinary tract, and gums.
   - Prevention: Control blood sugar levels, practice good hygiene, keep skin clean and dry, inspect skin for cuts or wounds, maintain oral hygiene, get recommended vaccinations, and seek prompt medical attention for any signs of infection.

By implementing these preventive strategies and actively managing your diabetes, you can reduce the risk of complications and maintain optimal health and well-being. Remember to work closely with your healthcare team to develop a personalized diabetes management plan that addresses your individual needs and helps you achieve your health goals.

- Importance of Regular Check-Ups

Regular check-ups are essential for individuals with diabetes to monitor their health, assess their diabetes management, and detect any potential complications early. Here are some reasons why regular check-ups are important for people with diabetes:

1. Monitoring Blood Sugar Levels:
   - Regular check-ups allow healthcare providers to monitor your blood sugar levels through blood tests such as A1c tests and fasting blood glucose tests. Monitoring blood sugar levels helps assess how well your diabetes is being managed and whether adjustments to your treatment plan are needed.

2. Assessing Diabetes Management:
   - Healthcare providers can evaluate your diabetes management strategies during check-ups, including medication adherence, dietary habits, physical activity levels, and self-monitoring practices. They can offer

guidance, support, and education to help you optimize your diabetes management.

3. Detecting Complications Early:
   - Regular check-ups enable healthcare providers to screen for and detect diabetes-related complications early, before they cause significant harm. This may include screenings for conditions such as diabetic retinopathy, nephropathy, neuropathy, cardiovascular disease, and foot problems.

4. Managing Risk Factors:
   - Healthcare providers can assess and manage risk factors for complications associated with diabetes, such as high blood pressure, high cholesterol, obesity, smoking, and sedentary lifestyle. They can offer guidance on lifestyle modifications, prescribe medications, and refer you to specialists as needed to reduce these risk factors.

5. Preventive Care and Vaccinations:
   - Regular check-ups provide opportunities for preventive care, including vaccinations to reduce the

risk of infections and complications. Healthcare providers may recommend vaccinations such as influenza (flu), pneumococcal, and hepatitis B vaccines to protect against infections that can be more severe in individuals with diabetes.

6. Medication Management:
   - Healthcare providers can review your medication regimen during check-ups, including diabetes medications, insulin therapy, and medications for managing comorbid conditions such as hypertension, dyslipidemia, and cardiovascular disease. They can adjust medication doses, prescribe new medications, or address any concerns or side effects.

7. Education and Support:
   - Regular check-ups provide opportunities for education and support to help you better understand your diabetes, develop self-management skills, and address any questions or concerns you may have. Healthcare providers can offer guidance on nutrition, physical activity, stress management, and coping strategies for living with diabetes.

8. Tracking Progress and Goal Setting:

   - Check-ups allow you to track your progress in managing diabetes and achieving health goals over time. Healthcare providers can review your goals, celebrate successes, identify areas for improvement, and adjust your treatment plan as needed to support your ongoing health and well-being.

9. Building a Strong Patient-Provider Relationship:

   - Regular check-ups help build a strong relationship between you and your healthcare provider based on trust, communication, and collaboration. A supportive and collaborative relationship with your healthcare team can enhance your motivation, engagement, and satisfaction with diabetes care.

10. Empowering Self-Management:

   - Check-ups empower you to take an active role in managing your diabetes and advocating for your health. By participating in regular check-ups, asking questions, sharing concerns, and working collaboratively with your healthcare team, you can make informed decisions and take control of your diabetes management.

Overall, regular check-ups are essential for optimizing diabetes management, preventing complications, and promoting long-term health and well-being. Make sure to schedule and attend regular check-ups with your healthcare provider as recommended to receive comprehensive care and support for your diabetes.

3.4 Navigating Social Situations

Navigating social situations with diabetes requires planning, communication, and confidence. Here are some tips to help you manage diabetes effectively in social settings:

1. Be Prepared:
  - Before attending social events, pack essential diabetes supplies such as blood glucose meter, testing strips, insulin, medications, snacks, and emergency supplies. Carry them with you in a discreet bag or pouch for easy access.

2. Communicate Openly:

   - Inform close friends, family members, and trusted companions about your diabetes and how they can support you. Explain any specific needs or concerns you may have, such as dietary restrictions or the need for breaks to check blood sugar levels or administer insulin.

3. Plan Ahead for Meals:

   - If you're attending an event with food, inquire about the menu in advance to make informed choices that align with your dietary preferences and diabetes management goals. Consider bringing a healthy dish or snack to share, ensuring there are options that suit your needs.

4. Monitor Blood Sugar Levels:

   - Regularly monitor your blood sugar levels during social gatherings, especially if there are changes in your routine, physical activity, or food intake. Check your blood sugar discreetly and respond promptly to any fluctuations to avoid hypoglycemia or hyperglycemia.

5. Manage Alcohol Intake:

  - If you choose to consume alcohol, do so in moderation and be mindful of its effects on blood sugar levels. Opt for lower-carbohydrate alcoholic beverages, alternate alcoholic drinks with water, and never drink on an empty stomach. Monitor your blood sugar levels closely and avoid excessive drinking.

6. Stay Active:

  - Incorporate physical activity into social activities whenever possible, such as going for a walk, dancing, or playing outdoor games. Staying active helps regulate blood sugar levels, promotes overall health, and enhances enjoyment of social gatherings.

7. Handle Peer Pressure Gracefully:

  - Be prepared to handle peer pressure or well-meaning but misguided advice about diabetes management. Politely assert your preferences and boundaries, educate others about diabetes when appropriate, and advocate for your health needs with confidence.

8. Be Flexible and Adaptive:

- Remain flexible and adaptive in managing diabetes in social situations, as unexpected changes or challenges may arise. Have backup plans in place, such as extra snacks, alternative meal options, or adjustments to your medication regimen, to navigate unforeseen circumstances.

9. Educate Others:
   - Take opportunities to educate friends, family members, and acquaintances about diabetes, dispel myths or misconceptions, and promote awareness and understanding. By sharing your experiences and knowledge, you can foster a supportive and inclusive environment.

10. Prioritize Self-Care:
   - Prioritize self-care and advocate for your health needs during social events. Listen to your body, take breaks when necessary, and prioritize activities that promote relaxation and well-being. Don't hesitate to excuse yourself from situations that feel overwhelming or uncomfortable.

By following these tips and strategies, you can navigate social situations with confidence, enjoy meaningful connections with others, and effectively manage diabetes while maintaining your overall health and well-being. Remember that you are not alone, and support is available to help you thrive in social settings with diabetes.

- Eating Out and Social Events

Managing diabetes while eating out and attending social events requires planning, flexibility, and mindful choices. Here are some tips to help you navigate these situations successfully:

1. Plan Ahead:
   - Review the menu of the restaurant or event venue in advance, if possible, to identify healthy options that align with your diabetes management goals. Look for dishes that are grilled, baked, steamed, or roasted, and opt for lean protein sources, vegetables, whole grains, and foods lower in saturated fats and added sugars.

2. Portion Control:

   - Pay attention to portion sizes and avoid oversized servings, which can lead to spikes in blood sugar levels. Consider sharing meals with a dining companion or requesting a half-sized portion to help manage portion control.

3. Choose Healthy Options:

   - Select nutrient-dense foods that are high in fiber, vitamins, and minerals, and low in refined carbohydrates and unhealthy fats. Choose salads, grilled or baked meats, seafood, vegetables, whole grains, and legumes as main options.

4. Modify Your Meal:

   - Don't hesitate to ask for modifications or substitutions to accommodate your dietary preferences and diabetes management needs. Request dressings, sauces, or condiments on the side, substitute starchy sides with extra vegetables or a salad, and choose water or unsweetened beverages instead of sugary drinks.

5. Monitor Carbohydrate Intake:

- Be mindful of carbohydrate-rich foods such as bread, rice, pasta, potatoes, and desserts, which can impact blood sugar levels. Opt for smaller portions of these foods or choose lower-carb alternatives when possible.

6. Control Your Portions:

   - Control your portions by using visual cues or portion control techniques, such as using smaller plates, dividing your plate into sections for protein, vegetables, and grains, and avoiding going back for seconds.

7. Monitor Blood Sugar Levels:

   - Monitor your blood sugar levels before, during, and after eating out or attending social events, especially if you're trying new foods or eating larger meals than usual. Be prepared to make adjustments to your insulin or medication doses as needed based on your blood sugar readings.

8. Be Mindful of Alcohol Intake:

   If you decide to consume alcohol, remember to drink it in moderation and be aware of how it affects your blood sugar levels. Choose lower-carbohydrate alcoholic beverages, alternate alcoholic drinks with water, and monitor your blood sugar levels closely to avoid hypoglycemia.

9. Stay Active:
   - Incorporate physical activity into social events whenever possible, such as taking a walk after a meal or dancing at a party. Staying active helps regulate blood sugar levels, promotes digestion, and supports overall health.

10. Plan for Desserts:
   - If you want to enjoy dessert, plan ahead by making smart choices and managing portion sizes. Consider sharing a dessert with a friend, opting for fruit-based desserts, or choosing smaller portions of your favorite treats.

By planning ahead, making mindful choices, monitoring your blood sugar levels, and advocating for your health needs, you can enjoy eating out and attending social events while effectively managing diabetes. Remember to prioritize balance, moderation, and self-care to support your overall well-being.

- Traveling with Diabetes

Traveling with diabetes requires careful planning and preparation to ensure you manage your condition effectively while away from home. Here are some tips to help you travel safely with diabetes:

1. Consult Your Healthcare Provider:
   - Before your trip, schedule a visit with your healthcare provider to discuss your travel plans, review your diabetes management strategies, and address any concerns or questions you may have. Make sure your diabetes is well-controlled before traveling.

2. Pack Sufficient Supplies:
   - Pack all necessary diabetes supplies, including blood glucose meters, testing strips, lancets, insulin, syringes or insulin pens, medications, glucose tablets or snacks

for treating low blood sugar, and a glucagon emergency
kit. In case of emergencies or unanticipated delays,
carry additional supplies.

3. Carry Prescriptions and Documentation:
   - Carry a list of your medications, doses, and
prescribing healthcare provider's contact information,
as well as a prescription for insulin or other
medications. Keep these documents with you in case you
need to refill prescriptions or explain your medical
needs to healthcare providers or security personnel.

4. Organize Supplies for Travel:
   - Organize your diabetes supplies in a clear,
waterproof bag or case to keep them organized and
easily accessible during travel. Pack supplies in your
carry-on luggage to avoid loss or damage, and store
insulin and medications in a cooler bag with ice packs to
maintain temperature stability.

5. Plan for Time Zone Changes:
   - If traveling across multiple time zones, adjust your
insulin dosing schedule accordingly to account for

changes in meal times and basal insulin requirements. Work with your healthcare provider to develop a plan for adjusting insulin doses during travel, and monitor your blood sugar levels closely during the transition period.

6. Monitor Blood Sugar Levels Regularly:
   - Monitor your blood sugar levels more frequently than usual during travel, especially if your routine is disrupted or you're experiencing changes in activity levels, diet, or stress. Carry a blood glucose meter and testing supplies with you at all times, and check your blood sugar before meals, snacks, and bedtime.

7. Stay Hydrated and Eat Regularly:
   - Stay hydrated by drinking plenty of water throughout your journey, as dehydration can affect blood sugar levels. Eat regular, balanced meals and snacks to maintain stable blood sugar levels and provide energy for travel activities.

8. Be Prepared for Emergencies:

- Familiarize yourself with the signs and symptoms of hypoglycemia (low blood sugar) and hyperglycemia (high blood sugar), and know how to respond to emergencies. Carry fast-acting carbohydrates such as glucose tablets, juice, or candy to treat low blood sugar, and have a plan for accessing medical care if needed.

9. Wear Medical Identification:
   - Wear a medical identification bracelet or necklace that indicates you have diabetes, along with any other relevant medical conditions or allergies. This can alert others to your medical needs in case of an emergency.

10. Research Healthcare Resources:
   - Research healthcare resources at your destination, including nearby hospitals, clinics, pharmacies, and diabetes specialists. Familiarize yourself with local emergency numbers and healthcare practices to ensure prompt access to medical care if needed.

By following these tips and planning ahead, you can travel safely and confidently with diabetes, allowing you to enjoy your trip while effectively managing your condition. Remember to prioritize self-care, monitor your blood sugar levels regularly, and seek medical assistance if you experience any diabetes-related complications during your travels.

Chapter 4:

Advanced Topics in Diabetes Care

4.1 Understanding the Latest Research

Understanding the latest research in diabetes can provide valuable insights into advancements in treatment, management strategies, and potential breakthroughs in the field. Here are some key areas of research in diabetes:

1. Genetics and Risk Factors:

- Researchers are studying the genetic factors that contribute to the development of type 1 and type 2 diabetes, as well as genetic predispositions for complications such as diabetic retinopathy, nephropathy, and neuropathy. Understanding the genetic basis of diabetes can help identify individuals at higher risk and inform personalized treatment approaches.

2. Beta Cell Regeneration:
   - Scientists are exploring approaches to regenerate or protect pancreatic beta cells, which produce insulin and are often damaged or destroyed in individuals with diabetes. Regenerative medicine techniques, such as stem cell therapy and beta cell transplantation, show promise for restoring insulin production and improving blood sugar control.

3. Artificial Pancreas Systems:
   - Research continues on the development and refinement of artificial pancreas systems, which combine continuous glucose monitoring (CGM) devices with insulin pumps to automate insulin delivery and

optimize blood sugar control. These systems aim to mimic the function of a healthy pancreas and reduce the burden of diabetes management for individuals with type 1 diabetes.

4. Immunotherapy and Immunomodulation:
   - Immunotherapy approaches are being investigated to prevent or reverse autoimmune destruction of pancreatic beta cells in type 1 diabetes. Immunomodulatory agents, such as monoclonal antibodies and immune checkpoint inhibitors, are being studied to modulate the immune response and preserve beta cell function.

5. Precision Medicine:
   - Researchers are exploring the use of precision medicine approaches to tailor diabetes treatment and management strategies to individual characteristics, including genetic, metabolic, and lifestyle factors. Personalized interventions, such as pharmacogenomics-guided therapy and lifestyle interventions based on behavioral profiling, aim to optimize outcomes and reduce the risk of complications.

6. Continuous Glucose Monitoring (CGM) Technology:
   - Advances in CGM technology are enhancing the accuracy, reliability, and usability of glucose monitoring devices, allowing individuals with diabetes to track their blood sugar levels in real-time and make well-informed decisions regarding food, exercise, and insulin dosage. Research is ongoing to further improve CGM accuracy, reduce sensor wear time, and integrate CGM data with automated insulin delivery systems.

7. Lifestyle Interventions:
   - Studies continue to investigate the impact of lifestyle interventions, including diet, exercise, weight management, and behavioral counseling, on diabetes prevention and management. Research is exploring novel approaches to promote sustainable behavior change, optimize dietary patterns, and increase physical activity levels to prevent or delay the onset of type 2 diabetes and improve outcomes for individuals with diabetes.

8. Pharmacotherapy and Novel Therapeutics:

- Research efforts are focused on developing new classes of diabetes medications, including oral antidiabetic agents, injectable therapies, and combination therapies, with improved efficacy, safety, and tolerability profiles. Novel therapeutic targets, such as incretin-based therapies, sodium-glucose cotransporter 2 (SGLT2) inhibitors, and glucagon-like peptide 1 (GLP-1) receptor agonists, are being explored to address unmet needs in diabetes management.

9. Digital Health and Telemedicine:
  - The integration of digital health technologies, telemedicine platforms, and mobile health applications into diabetes care is expanding access to education, self-management tools, remote monitoring, and virtual healthcare services. Research is evaluating the effectiveness and feasibility of digital interventions for improving diabetes outcomes and enhancing patient engagement and empowerment.

10. Health Equity and Access to Care:
  - Researchers are examining disparities in diabetes prevalence, outcomes, and access to care based on

socioeconomic status, race, ethnicity, geography, and other factors. Efforts to address health equity in diabetes care aim to reduce disparities, improve access to affordable healthcare services and medications, and promote culturally sensitive and patient-centered approaches to diabetes management.

Staying informed about the latest research findings in diabetes can empower individuals with diabetes, healthcare providers, and policymakers to make evidence-based decisions, advance scientific knowledge, and improve outcomes for people living with diabetes. Collaborative efforts across research disciplines, healthcare sectors, and patient advocacy groups are essential for translating research discoveries into clinical practice and public health initiatives that benefit individuals and communities affected by diabetes.

- Innovations in Diabetes Treatment

Innovations in diabetes treatment are revolutionizing the way diabetes is managed, offering new options for improving blood sugar control, reducing complications, and enhancing quality of life for individuals with diabetes. Here are some notable innovations in diabetes treatment:

1. Continuous Glucose Monitoring (CGM) Systems:
   - CGM systems use sensors to continuously monitor glucose levels in interstitial fluid, providing real-time data on blood sugar trends and patterns. These devices offer insights into glucose fluctuations, help identify hypoglycemia and hyperglycemia episodes, and support informed decision-making regarding insulin dosing, diet, and physical activity.

2. Insulin Delivery Systems:
   - Advanced insulin delivery systems, such as insulin pumps and patch pumps, provide precise and customizable insulin dosing, reducing the need for multiple daily injections and improving insulin delivery accuracy. Integrated insulin pump systems with CGM technology offer hybrid closed-loop systems, also known as artificial pancreas systems, which automate insulin delivery based on CGM data.

3. Injectable Therapies:

 - Injectable therapies for diabetes management, including glucagon-like peptide 1 (GLP-1) receptor agonists and sodium-glucose cotransporter 2 (SGLT2) inhibitors, offer additional options for blood sugar control and cardiovascular risk reduction. These medications work by stimulating insulin secretion, suppressing glucagon production, promoting weight loss, and reducing blood pressure and cardiovascular events.

4. Oral Antidiabetic Agents:

 - Oral antidiabetic agents, such as dipeptidyl peptidase 4 (DPP-4) inhibitors, sodium-glucose cotransporter 2 (SGLT2) inhibitors, and biguanides, provide oral alternatives to injectable insulin therapy for individuals with type 2 diabetes. These medications improve glycemic control, lower blood sugar levels, and reduce the risk of cardiovascular complications.

5. Closed-Loop Insulin Delivery Systems:

- Closed-loop insulin delivery systems, also known as artificial pancreas systems, combine CGM technology with insulin pumps to automate insulin delivery based on real-time glucose readings. These systems adjust insulin dosing dynamically to maintain blood sugar levels within target ranges, reducing the risk of hypoglycemia and hyperglycemia.

6. Implantable Devices:
  - Implantable devices, such as continuous glucose monitors (CGMs) and insulin pumps, offer long-term glucose monitoring and insulin delivery solutions for individuals with diabetes. Implantable CGM sensors provide continuous glucose monitoring without the need for external devices, while implantable insulin pumps deliver insulin directly into the body through subcutaneous infusion.

7. Gene Therapy and Regenerative Medicine:
  - Gene therapy and regenerative medicine approaches are being explored to regenerate or protect pancreatic beta cells, restore insulin production, and reverse autoimmune destruction in type 1 diabetes. These

innovative therapies aim to address the underlying causes of diabetes and offer potential cures or long-term remission for the disease.

8. Telemedicine and Digital Health Solutions:
   - Telemedicine platforms, mobile health applications, and digital health solutions are transforming diabetes care by expanding access to remote monitoring, virtual consultations, telehealth services, and patient education resources. These technologies enhance communication between patients and healthcare providers, improve diabetes self-management, and support personalized treatment plans.

9. Personalized Medicine and Precision Therapy:
   - Personalized medicine approaches, including pharmacogenomics, biomarker testing, and genetic profiling, enable tailored treatment plans based on individual characteristics, such as genetic, metabolic, and lifestyle factors. Precision therapy aims to optimize diabetes management by matching patients with the most effective medications and interventions for their unique needs and preferences.

10. Lifestyle Interventions and Behavioral Health
Support:

 - Lifestyle interventions, including diet, exercise, weight management, and behavioral counseling, play a critical role in diabetes prevention and management. Innovative programs and technologies support behavior change, promote healthy habits, and address psychosocial factors that influence diabetes outcomes, such as stress, depression, and social support.

These innovations in diabetes treatment represent significant advancements in diabetes care, offering new opportunities for personalized, effective, and patient-centered approaches to managing diabetes and improving quality of life for individuals with the condition. By leveraging these innovative therapies and technologies, healthcare providers and individuals with diabetes can optimize treatment outcomes, reduce complications, and empower patients to live well with diabetes.

- Future Directions in Diabetes Care

Future directions in diabetes care are guided by ongoing research, technological advancements, and evolving healthcare practices aimed at improving outcomes, enhancing patient experience, and reducing the burden of diabetes on individuals and healthcare systems. Here are some potential future directions in diabetes care:

1. Precision Medicine and Personalized Treatment:
   - Precision medicine approaches will continue to evolve, leveraging genetic, metabolic, and lifestyle data to tailor diabetes treatment and management strategies to individual characteristics and preferences. Personalized treatment plans will optimize outcomes by matching patients with the most effective medications, interventions, and lifestyle modifications for their unique needs.

2. Artificial Intelligence and Predictive Analytics:

- Artificial intelligence (AI) and machine learning algorithms will play a growing role in diabetes care, analyzing large datasets, identifying patterns, and predicting individualized risk profiles for diabetes complications, treatment responses, and health outcomes. Predictive analytics will enable early intervention and proactive management to prevent complications and optimize long-term health.

3. Digital Health Technologies and Telemedicine:
  - Digital health technologies, telemedicine platforms, and mobile health applications will expand access to diabetes care, offering remote monitoring, virtual consultations, telehealth services, and self-management tools. These technologies will enhance communication between patients and healthcare providers, improve adherence to treatment plans, and empower individuals to take control of their diabetes management.

4. Continuous Glucose Monitoring (CGM) and Closed-Loop Systems:
  - Continuous glucose monitoring (CGM) systems and closed-loop insulin delivery systems will become more

sophisticated and widely adopted, offering real-time data on blood sugar trends and automating insulin dosing based on CGM readings. These systems will optimize blood sugar control, reduce the risk of hypoglycemia and hyperglycemia, and enhance quality of life for individuals with diabetes.

5. Regenerative Medicine and Beta Cell Replacement Therapy:
   - Regenerative medicine approaches and beta cell replacement therapies hold promise for restoring insulin production and reversing diabetes in individuals with type 1 diabetes. Stem cell therapy, beta cell transplantation, and gene editing techniques will continue to be explored as potential cures or long-term treatments for the disease.

6. Multidisciplinary Care and Integrated Health Models:
   - Multidisciplinary care models and integrated health systems will facilitate collaborative approaches to diabetes management, involving healthcare providers, specialists, educators, pharmacists, and allied health professionals. Coordinated care delivery will address the

complex needs of individuals with diabetes, promote holistic health and well-being, and improve treatment adherence and outcomes.

7. Patient-Centered Care and Shared Decision-Making:
  - Patient-centered care models and shared decision-making processes will prioritize individual preferences, values, and goals in diabetes treatment planning. Empowering patients to actively participate in their care, express their needs, and make informed decisions will enhance engagement, satisfaction, and adherence to treatment plans.

8. Health Equity and Access to Care:
  - Efforts to address health equity in diabetes care will focus on reducing disparities in diabetes prevalence, outcomes, and access to care based on socioeconomic status, race, ethnicity, geography, and other factors. Culturally sensitive and patient-centered approaches will promote inclusivity, diversity, and equity in diabetes management.

9. Prevention and Early Intervention:

- Emphasis will be placed on prevention and early intervention strategies to reduce the incidence of type 2 diabetes and delay the progression of prediabetes to diabetes. Population-based interventions, community outreach programs, and public health initiatives will promote healthy lifestyles, encourage screening and early detection, and target modifiable risk factors for diabetes.

10. Research and Innovation:
   - Ongoing research and innovation will drive advancements in diabetes care, including novel therapeutic targets, innovative treatment modalities, and breakthrough technologies. Collaborative efforts across research disciplines, healthcare sectors, and patient advocacy groups will accelerate progress towards preventing, managing, and ultimately curing diabetes.

These future directions in diabetes care reflect a commitment to continuous improvement, innovation, and patient-centered approaches that prioritize the needs and preferences of individuals with diabetes. By embracing these advancements and working collaboratively, healthcare providers, researchers, policymakers, and individuals with diabetes can achieve better outcomes, reduce complications, and enhance quality of life for everyone affected by diabetes.

4.2 Technological Tools for Diabetes Management

Technological tools for diabetes management have revolutionized the way individuals with diabetes monitor their blood sugar levels, administer insulin, track their health data, and make informed decisions about their care. Here are some key technological tools used in diabetes management:

1. Continuous Glucose Monitoring (CGM) Systems:
   - CGM systems use sensors inserted under the skin to continuously monitor glucose levels in interstitial fluid. These systems provide real-time data on blood sugar trends, alert users to high and low glucose levels, and track glucose patterns over time. CGM devices help

individuals with diabetes make informed decisions about insulin dosing, diet, and physical activity to optimize blood sugar control.

2. Insulin Pumps:
   - Insulin pumps are small, wearable devices that deliver insulin continuously through a catheter inserted under the skin. Insulin pumps provide precise and customizable insulin dosing, allowing users to program basal rates, bolus doses, and correction factors to meet their individual insulin needs. Pump therapy offers flexibility, convenience, and improved blood sugar control for individuals with diabetes.

3. Automated Insulin Delivery Systems:
   - Automated insulin delivery systems, also known as closed-loop systems or artificial pancreas systems, combine CGM technology with insulin pumps to automate insulin delivery based on real-time glucose readings. These systems adjust insulin dosing dynamically to maintain blood sugar levels within target ranges, reducing the risk of hypoglycemia and hyperglycemia.

4. Mobile Apps and Digital Platforms:

   - Mobile apps and digital platforms offer a variety of tools and resources for diabetes management, including glucose tracking, meal planning, medication reminders, exercise tracking, and educational content. These apps enable users to monitor their health data, set goals, track progress, and share information with healthcare providers for personalized feedback and support.

5. Telemedicine and Virtual Care:

   - Telemedicine platforms and virtual care services provide remote access to healthcare providers, allowing individuals with diabetes to receive consultations, monitoring, and support from the comfort of their own homes. Telemedicine appointments facilitate regular check-ups, medication management, and diabetes education without the need for in-person visits.

6. Smart Insulin Pens:

   - Smart insulin pens are pen-like devices equipped with Bluetooth technology that track insulin doses, injection times, and blood sugar readings. These devices

sync with mobile apps to provide users with real-time
feedback on insulin usage, dose history, and adherence
to treatment plans. Smart pens help users manage their
insulin therapy more effectively and improve medication
adherence.

7. Wearable Health Devices:
  - Wearable health devices, such as fitness trackers,
smartwatches, and wearable sensors, offer additional
monitoring capabilities for individuals with diabetes.
These devices track physical activity, sleep patterns,
heart rate, and other health metrics, providing insights
into overall health and lifestyle factors that impact blood
sugar control.

8. Remote Patient Monitoring Systems:
  - Remote patient monitoring systems allow healthcare
providers to remotely monitor patients' health data,
including blood sugar levels, medication adherence, and
treatment outcomes. These systems enable proactive
intervention, timely adjustments to treatment plans, and
early detection of potential complications, improving
the quality of care for individuals with diabetes.

9. Artificial Intelligence and Predictive Analytics:
   - Artificial intelligence (AI) algorithms and predictive analytics tools analyze large datasets of health information to identify patterns, predict future trends, and personalize diabetes management strategies. AI-powered decision support systems offer insights into optimal insulin dosing, dietary choices, and lifestyle modifications based on individual characteristics and glucose patterns.

10. Online Support Communities and Peer Networks:
   - Online support communities, social media groups, and peer networks provide a platform for individuals with diabetes to connect, share experiences, and exchange advice and encouragement. These virtual communities offer emotional support, practical tips, and a sense of belonging for individuals navigating the challenges of diabetes management.

By leveraging these technological tools and resources, individuals with diabetes can take an active role in managing their condition, optimize blood sugar control, reduce the risk of complications, and improve overall health and well-being. Collaborative efforts between patients, healthcare providers, technology developers, and researchers will continue to drive innovation and advancement in diabetes management, empowering individuals to live well with diabetes.

- Apps and Devices

Certainly! Here's a breakdown of some popular apps and devices used in diabetes management:

Apps:

1. mySugr: This app allows users to track blood sugar levels, carbohydrates, insulin doses, and physical activity. It offers personalized insights, reminders, and reports to help users manage their diabetes effectively.

2. BG Monitor Diabetes: BG Monitor Diabetes enables users to log blood glucose readings, medications, meals,

and exercise. It provides customizable reports and trends to monitor diabetes management over time.

3. Glucose Buddy: Glucose Buddy tracks blood sugar levels, insulin doses, medications, meals, and physical activity. It offers data visualization, reminders, and sharing options for users and healthcare providers.

4. Diabetes:M: Diabetes:M serves as a comprehensive diabetes management tool, allowing users to track blood sugar levels, insulin doses, medications, meals, and exercise. It provides personalized insights, health tips, and educational content.

5. Carb Manager: Carb Manager helps users track carbohydrate intake, manage meal plans, and monitor nutrition. It offers a database of foods with nutritional information, recipes, and macro tracking features.

6. Fooducate: Fooducate helps users make healthier food choices by providing nutritional information, ingredient analysis, and product ratings. It offers personalized meal

recommendations and tracking tools for managing diabetes-friendly diets.

7. One Drop: One Drop offers personalized diabetes management plans, blood sugar tracking, medication reminders, and coaching support. It integrates with glucose meters, fitness trackers, and other health devices for comprehensive monitoring.

8. Diasend: Diasend allows users to sync data from various diabetes devices, including glucose meters, insulin pumps, and CGM systems. It provides comprehensive reports, data visualization, and remote monitoring for diabetes management.

9. Sugar Sense: Sugar Sense tracks blood sugar levels, carbohydrates, insulin doses, and medications. It offers personalized insights, reminders, and educational content to support diabetes self-management.

10. Glooko: Glooko enables users to sync data from diabetes devices, track blood sugar levels, medications, and lifestyle factors, and share information with

healthcare providers. It offers personalized analytics and coaching support for diabetes management.

Devices:

1. Continuous Glucose Monitors (CGMs): CGMs, such as Dexcom G6, Abbott FreeStyle Libre, and Medtronic Guardian Sensor, continuously monitor glucose levels in interstitial fluid and provide real-time data on blood sugar trends.

2. Insulin Pumps: Insulin pumps, like Medtronic MiniMed 670G, Tandem t:slim X2, and Omnipod DASH, deliver insulin continuously through a catheter inserted under the skin, allowing for precise and customizable insulin dosing.

3. Smart Insulin Pens: Smart insulin pens, such as InPen and Timesulin, track insulin doses, injection times, and blood sugar readings. They sync with mobile apps to provide real-time feedback on insulin usage and adherence.

4. Blood Glucose Meters: Blood glucose meters, such as Accu-Chek Guide, OneTouch Verio, and Contour Next One, measure blood sugar levels using small blood samples and provide accurate readings within seconds.

5. Ketone Meters: Ketone meters, like Keto Mojo and Precision Xtra, measure ketone levels in blood or urine to monitor ketosis in individuals following low-carb or ketogenic diets.

6. Activity Trackers: Activity trackers, such as Fitbit, Garmin, and Apple Watch, monitor physical activity, sleep patterns, heart rate, and calorie expenditure to support overall health and diabetes management.

7. Smart Scales: Smart scales, such as Withings Body+, FitTrack, and Etekcity, measure body weight, body composition, and other metrics to track progress and support weight management goals in individuals with diabetes.

8. Bluetooth Blood Pressure Monitors: Bluetooth blood pressure monitors, like Omron Evolv and QardioArm,

measure blood pressure levels and sync data with mobile apps for monitoring hypertension and cardiovascular health in individuals with diabetes.

9. Smart Thermometers: Smart thermometers, such as Kinsa Smart Thermometer and Withings Thermo, measure body temperature and provide insights into fever trends and illness management for individuals with diabetes.

10. Smart Kitchen Appliances: Smart kitchen appliances, like smart scales, air fryers, and pressure cookers, offer convenient and healthy cooking options for individuals with diabetes, supporting meal planning and management of diabetes-friendly diets.

These apps and devices offer valuable tools and resources for individuals with diabetes to monitor their health, manage their condition, and make informed decisions about their care. By incorporating these technologies into their diabetes management routines, individuals can optimize blood sugar control, reduce the risk of complications, and improve overall well-being.

- How Technology Can Help

Technology plays a crucial role in diabetes management, offering a wide range of tools and resources to help individuals monitor their blood sugar levels, track their health data, manage their medications, make informed decisions about their care, and connect with healthcare providers and support networks. Here are some ways technology can help:

1. Continuous Glucose Monitoring (CGM):
   - CGM systems provide real-time data on blood sugar levels, allowing individuals to monitor glucose trends, identify patterns, and make timely adjustments to their treatment plans. CGM devices alert users to high and low blood sugar levels, reducing the risk of hypo- and hyperglycemia and improving overall blood sugar control.

2. Insulin Delivery Systems:
   - Insulin pumps and smart insulin pens offer precise and customizable insulin dosing, helping individuals

with diabetes manage their insulin therapy more effectively. These devices automate insulin delivery, track insulin doses, and provide reminders to ensure adherence to treatment plans.

3. Mobile Apps and Digital Platforms:
   - Mobile apps and digital platforms offer a variety of tools and resources for diabetes management, including blood sugar tracking, medication reminders, meal planning, and educational content. These apps provide personalized insights, support behavior change, and facilitate communication with healthcare providers.

4. Telemedicine and Virtual Care:
   - Telemedicine platforms and virtual care services enable individuals with diabetes to receive consultations, monitoring, and support from healthcare providers remotely. Telemedicine appointments offer convenient access to care, reduce the need for in-person visits, and promote continuity of care for individuals managing chronic conditions like diabetes.

5. Remote Patient Monitoring:

- Remote patient monitoring systems allow healthcare providers to remotely monitor patients' health data, including blood sugar levels, medication adherence, and treatment outcomes. These systems enable proactive intervention, timely adjustments to treatment plans, and early detection of potential complications, improving the quality of care for individuals with diabetes.

6. Artificial Intelligence and Predictive Analytics:
   - Artificial intelligence (AI) algorithms and predictive analytics tools analyze health data to identify patterns, predict future trends, and personalize diabetes management strategies. AI-powered decision support systems offer insights into optimal treatment approaches, help optimize blood sugar control, and reduce the risk of complications.

7. Wearable Health Devices:
 - Wearable health devices, such as fitness trackers, smartwatches, and wearable sensors, provide additional monitoring capabilities for individuals with diabetes. These devices track physical activity, sleep patterns, heart rate, and other health metrics, offering insights

into overall health and lifestyle factors that impact blood sugar control.

8. Smart Kitchen Appliances:
  - Smart kitchen appliances offer convenient and healthy cooking options for individuals with diabetes, supporting meal planning and management of diabetes-friendly diets. These appliances provide recipes, nutritional information, and portion control guidance to help individuals make healthier food choices and maintain blood sugar control.

9. Online Support Communities:
  - Online support communities, social media groups, and peer networks provide a platform for individuals with diabetes to connect, share experiences, and exchange advice and encouragement. These virtual communities offer emotional support, practical tips, and a sense of belonging for individuals navigating the challenges of diabetes management.

10. Health Education and Self-Management Tools:

- Health education resources and self-management tools empower individuals with diabetes to learn about their condition, develop self-care skills, and take an active role in managing their health. These resources provide information on diabetes management, lifestyle modifications, medication adherence, and coping strategies for living well with diabetes.

Overall, technology enhances diabetes management by providing individuals with access to information, tools, and support resources that empower them to make informed decisions, optimize blood sugar control, reduce the risk of complications, and improve their quality of life. By leveraging these technological advancements, individuals with diabetes can effectively manage their condition and achieve better health outcomes.

4.3 Personalized Medicine

Personalized medicine, also known as precision medicine, is an approach to healthcare that involves tailoring medical treatment and interventions to individual characteristics, including genetic, genomic, environmental, and lifestyle factors. The goal of personalized medicine is to optimize treatment outcomes, improve patient satisfaction, and reduce the risk of adverse effects by considering the unique needs and characteristics of each patient.

In the context of diabetes management, personalized medicine encompasses a range of approaches aimed at tailoring treatment plans and interventions to individual characteristics and preferences. Here are some key aspects of personalized medicine in diabetes care:

1. Genetic and Genomic Testing:
  - Genetic and genomic testing can identify genetic variants and biomarkers associated with diabetes risk, treatment response, and complications. By analyzing an individual's genetic profile, healthcare providers can personalize treatment plans and interventions to target

specific genetic factors that influence diabetes management.

2. Pharmacogenomics:
   - Pharmacogenomics examines how genetic variations affect an individual's response to medications. By analyzing genetic markers related to drug metabolism, efficacy, and safety, healthcare providers can tailor medication selection and dosing to optimize therapeutic outcomes and minimize the risk of adverse drug reactions in individuals with diabetes.

3. Lifestyle and Behavioral Factors:
   - Personalized medicine considers lifestyle and behavioral factors, such as diet, exercise, stress management, and sleep habits, that impact diabetes management. Healthcare providers work with patients to develop personalized lifestyle interventions and behavior change strategies tailored to their individual preferences, cultural background, and social context.

4. Risk Stratification and Prevention:

- Personalized medicine involves risk stratification to identify individuals at higher risk of developing diabetes or diabetes-related complications. By assessing individual risk factors, healthcare providers can implement targeted preventive measures, such as lifestyle modifications, screening tests, and early intervention programs, to reduce the risk of diabetes onset and progression.

5. Treatment Selection and Optimization:
  - Personalized medicine guides treatment selection and optimization based on individual characteristics, including disease severity, comorbidities, medication history, and treatment preferences. Healthcare providers tailor treatment plans to meet the specific needs and goals of each patient, adjusting medication regimens, insulin dosing strategies, and adjunctive therapies as needed.

6. Continuous Monitoring and Data Integration:
  - Personalized medicine incorporates continuous monitoring of health data, including blood sugar levels, medication adherence, lifestyle factors, and treatment

outcomes. Healthcare providers use data integration platforms and digital health technologies to track patient progress, identify trends, and make data-driven decisions to optimize diabetes management.

7. Shared Decision-Making and Patient Engagement:
   - Personalized medicine emphasizes shared decision-making and patient engagement in diabetes care. Healthcare professionals work together with patients to create individualized treatment programs that complement their objectives, values, and preferences. Patients are empowered to actively participate in their care, make informed decisions, and take ownership of their health.

8. Health Equity and Cultural Competence:
   - Personalized medicine acknowledges the importance of health equity and cultural competence in diabetes care. Healthcare providers recognize and address disparities in diabetes prevalence, outcomes, and access to care based on socioeconomic status, race, ethnicity, and other factors. Culturally sensitive and patient-

centered approaches promote inclusivity, diversity, and equity in diabetes management.

Overall, personalized medicine holds promise for improving diabetes care by tailoring treatment plans and interventions to individual characteristics, preferences, and needs. By embracing personalized approaches to diabetes management, healthcare providers can optimize treatment outcomes, enhance patient satisfaction, and empower individuals to achieve better health and well-being.

- **Tailoring Treatment to Individual Needs**

Tailoring treatment to individual needs is a cornerstone of effective diabetes management, as it recognizes that each person's experience with diabetes is unique and requires personalized approaches to achieve optimal outcomes. Here are some key principles and strategies for tailoring treatment to individual needs in diabetes care:

1. Comprehensive Assessment:

- Conduct a thorough assessment of each individual's medical history, including diabetes duration, complications, comorbidities, medication history, lifestyle factors, and psychosocial context. Understanding the individual's unique circumstances and preferences forms the basis for personalized treatment planning.

2. Individualized Treatment Goals:
- Collaborate with the individual to establish personalized treatment goals that are realistic, achievable, and aligned with their priorities and preferences. Tailor glycemic targets, blood pressure goals, lipid levels, and other treatment objectives to reflect the individual's age, health status, life stage, and quality of life considerations.

3. Lifestyle Modification:
- Customize lifestyle interventions, including diet, exercise, weight management, and stress reduction strategies, to meet the individual's specific needs and preferences. Consider cultural background, socioeconomic factors, food preferences, physical

activity preferences, and barriers to behavior change when designing personalized lifestyle plans.

4. Medication Selection and Adjustment:
  - Individualize medication selection based on factors such as diabetes type, disease severity, treatment history, renal function, cardiovascular risk, and medication tolerability. Tailor medication regimens to address the individual's unique needs and goals, adjusting dosages, formulations, and combinations as needed to optimize treatment efficacy and safety.

5. Patient Education and Empowerment:
  - Provide tailored patient education and support to empower individuals with the knowledge, skills, and confidence to manage their diabetes effectively. Address the individual's learning style, health literacy level, cultural beliefs, and preferences when delivering educational materials and self-management resources.

6. Continuous Monitoring and Feedback:
  - Implement regular monitoring of blood sugar levels, medication adherence, lifestyle behaviors, and treatment

outcomes to track progress and identify areas for intervention. Provide personalized feedback, support, and guidance based on the individual's data and preferences to facilitate ongoing self-management and behavior change.

7. Shared Decision-Making and Communication:
   - Engage in shared decision-making with the individual to involve them in treatment planning, goal setting, and care decisions. Foster open, transparent communication, listen to the individual's concerns and preferences, and respect their autonomy and choices in managing their diabetes.

8. Psychosocial Support and Mental Health Care:
   - Address psychosocial factors, emotional well-being, and mental health concerns as integral components of diabetes care. Offer personalized support, counseling, and resources to help individuals cope with the emotional impact of diabetes, manage stress, address depression or anxiety symptoms, and build resilience.

9. Multidisciplinary Collaboration:

- Collaborate with a multidisciplinary team of healthcare providers, including physicians, nurses, dietitians, pharmacists, psychologists, and other specialists, to provide comprehensive, coordinated care that addresses the individual's diverse needs and concerns.

10. Long-Term Follow-Up and Continuity of Care:
  - Establish a long-term follow-up plan and continuity of care to ensure ongoing support, monitoring, and management of diabetes over time. Regularly reassess the individual's treatment plan, adjust interventions as needed, and maintain open lines of communication to promote sustained engagement and adherence.

By tailoring treatment to individual needs, healthcare providers can personalize diabetes care, optimize treatment outcomes, enhance patient satisfaction, and empower individuals to achieve better health and well-being. Customized approaches that consider the unique characteristics, preferences, and circumstances of each person with diabetes foster a collaborative and patient-centered approach to diabetes management.

- Genetic and Environmental Considerations

Genetic and environmental factors both play significant roles in the development, progression, and management of diabetes. Understanding how these factors interact can help healthcare providers tailor treatment plans and interventions to individual needs. Here's a closer look at genetic and environmental considerations in diabetes care:

Genetic Considerations:

1. **Genetic Predisposition:** Genetic predisposition plays a key role in the development of both type 1 and type 2 diabetes. Individuals with a family history of diabetes have a higher risk of developing the condition due to shared genetic susceptibility factors.

2. **Genetic Variants:** Specific genetic variants have been identified as risk factors for diabetes. For example, certain variants in genes such as TCF7L2, PPARG, KCNJ11, and HNF1A are associated with an increased

risk of type 2 diabetes, while variants in the HLA region are linked to an increased risk of type 1 diabetes.

3. **Monogenic Forms of Diabetes:** Monogenic forms of diabetes, such as maturity-onset diabetes of the young (MODY) and neonatal diabetes, are caused by mutations in a single gene. These genetic subtypes of diabetes often present with distinct clinical features and may require specific treatment approaches.

4. **Pharmacogenomics:** Pharmacogenomic factors influence an individual's response to diabetes medications. Genetic variations in drug metabolism enzymes, transporters, and receptors can affect medication efficacy, safety, and side effects, guiding personalized medication selection and dosing.

5. **Precision Medicine:** Precision medicine approaches leverage genetic testing and genomic analysis to personalize diabetes treatment plans. By identifying genetic variants and biomarkers associated with diabetes risk and treatment response, healthcare

providers can tailor interventions to individual genetic profiles.

Environmental Considerations:

1. **Lifestyle Factors:** Environmental factors, such as diet, physical activity, smoking, and stress, play significant roles in diabetes development and management. Unhealthy lifestyle behaviors, such as poor diet and sedentary habits, can contribute to insulin resistance, obesity, and metabolic dysfunction.

2. **Obesogenic Environment:** The obesogenic environment, characterized by easy access to high-calorie, low-nutrient foods and sedentary lifestyles, contributes to the rising prevalence of obesity and type 2 diabetes. Environmental interventions that promote healthy eating, active living, and built environment changes can help mitigate these risk factors.

3. **Socioeconomic Factors:** Socioeconomic factors, including income, education, employment, and access to healthcare, influence diabetes risk and outcomes.

Individuals from disadvantaged socioeconomic backgrounds are more likely to experience barriers to diabetes prevention, diagnosis, and management.

4. **Psychosocial Stress:** Psychosocial stressors, such as job strain, financial difficulties, trauma, and discrimination, can exacerbate diabetes risk and worsen glycemic control. Addressing psychosocial factors and providing support for stress management can improve diabetes outcomes and quality of life.

5. **Environmental Toxins:** Environmental toxins, such as air pollution, endocrine-disrupting chemicals, and heavy metals, may contribute to insulin resistance, inflammation, and metabolic dysfunction. Minimizing exposure to environmental toxins and promoting environmental policies that protect public health can help reduce diabetes risk.

Integration of Genetic and Environmental Factors:

Integrating genetic and environmental considerations in diabetes care involves assessing both individual susceptibility factors and modifiable lifestyle factors to develop personalized treatment plans. By addressing genetic predisposition, lifestyle behaviors, and environmental influences, healthcare providers can tailor interventions to target the root causes of diabetes and optimize treatment outcomes for each individual. This holistic approach to diabetes management recognizes the complex interplay between genetic and environmental factors and empowers individuals to take proactive steps towards better health and well-being.

4.4 Diabetes in Special Populations

Diabetes affects people from all walks of life, but certain populations face unique challenges and considerations in diabetes prevention, diagnosis, and management. Here are some special populations that healthcare providers should consider when addressing diabetes care:

1. Children and Adolescents:

- Pediatric diabetes, including type 1 diabetes and increasingly prevalent type 2 diabetes, requires specialized care tailored to the developmental stage and unique needs of children and adolescents. Management strategies must address growth and development, family dynamics, psychosocial factors, and transition to self-care as children transition into adulthood.

2. Older Adults:
  - Older adults with diabetes face distinct challenges related to aging, comorbidities, cognitive impairment, functional limitations, polypharmacy, and frailty. Diabetes management must consider individualized treatment goals, medication safety, geriatric syndromes, fall risk, and end-of-life care preferences in this population.

3. Pregnant Women:
  - Gestational diabetes mellitus (GDM) and pre-existing diabetes present risks to both maternal and fetal health during pregnancy. Comprehensive prenatal care involves screening, monitoring, and managing blood sugar levels to optimize pregnancy outcomes, reduce the

risk of maternal and neonatal complications, and promote long-term health for both mother and child.

4. Racial and Ethnic Minorities:
   - Racial and ethnic minorities, including African Americans, Hispanic/Latino Americans, Native Americans, and Asian Americans, have higher rates of diabetes prevalence, complications, and disparities in access to care. Culturally competent and community-based interventions are essential to address social determinants of health, reduce disparities, and promote health equity in diabetes care.

5. Socioeconomically Disadvantaged Populations:
   - Socioeconomically disadvantaged populations, including individuals with low income, limited education, inadequate health insurance, and food insecurity, face barriers to diabetes prevention, diagnosis, and management. Access to affordable healthcare, nutritious food, safe environments for physical activity, and social support services is critical to addressing disparities and improving health outcomes in underserved communities.

6. LGBTQ+ Individuals:
   - LGBTQ+ individuals may face unique challenges related to stigma, discrimination, mental health disparities, and barriers to healthcare access, which can impact diabetes risk and management. Culturally sensitive and affirming care that addresses the specific needs and concerns of LGBTQ+ individuals is essential to promote health and well-being in this population.

7. Individuals with Disabilities:
   - Individuals with disabilities, including physical, intellectual, developmental, and sensory disabilities, may experience barriers to diabetes self-management, healthcare access, and health literacy. Diabetes care must be adapted to accommodate individual abilities, communication preferences, assistive technologies, and support networks to promote autonomy and quality of life.

8. Rural and Remote Communities:
   - Rural and remote communities face challenges related to geographic isolation, limited healthcare

resources, transportation barriers, and workforce shortages, which can impact diabetes prevention, screening, and access to specialty care. Telemedicine, community health worker programs, mobile clinics, and telehealth initiatives can help bridge gaps in diabetes care and improve health outcomes in underserved areas.

9. Individuals with Mental Health Conditions:
   - Individuals with mental health conditions, such as depression, anxiety, bipolar disorder, schizophrenia, and eating disorders, are at higher risk of diabetes and may face challenges in diabetes self-management, medication adherence, and lifestyle modification. Integrated care models that address both physical and mental health needs are essential to provide comprehensive support and improve outcomes for this population.

10. Immigrant and Refugee Populations:
   - Immigrant and refugee populations may encounter cultural, linguistic, and structural barriers to diabetes care, including limited health literacy, language proficiency, cultural beliefs, and access to culturally

competent services. Culturally sensitive care, language interpretation services, community outreach, and navigation assistance can help address these barriers and promote health equity in immigrant and refugee communities.

By recognizing the diverse needs, experiences, and contexts of special populations affected by diabetes, healthcare providers can implement tailored interventions, culturally responsive care, and multidisciplinary approaches to promote health equity, improve outcomes, and enhance quality of life for all individuals living with diabetes.

- Children and Adolescents

Children and adolescents with diabetes require specialized care that considers their unique developmental, physical, emotional, and social needs. Here are some key considerations for healthcare providers when addressing diabetes care in this population:

1. Early Diagnosis and Education:
   - Early diagnosis of diabetes in children and adolescents is crucial for timely intervention and management. Healthcare providers should educate parents, caregivers, and school personnel about the signs and symptoms of diabetes and encourage prompt medical evaluation for any concerning symptoms.

2. Family-Centered Care:
   - Diabetes management in children and adolescents should involve a family-centered approach that engages parents, siblings, and other caregivers in the child's care. Collaborative decision-making, open communication, and shared responsibility for diabetes management help support the child's well-being and adherence to treatment plans.

3. Developmentally Appropriate Education:
   - Provide developmentally appropriate education and support to children and adolescents with diabetes,

considering their age, cognitive abilities, and level of understanding. Use child-friendly language, visual aids, and interactive tools to explain diabetes concepts, self-care tasks, and treatment goals in a way that is understandable and empowering.

4. Psychosocial Support:
   - Address the psychosocial impact of diabetes on children and adolescents, including stress, anxiety, depression, body image concerns, and social stigma. Offer counseling, peer support groups, and resources to help children and families cope with emotional challenges and build resilience in managing diabetes.

5. Transition to Self-Care:
   - Support children and adolescents with diabetes in gradually transitioning to self-care and independent management as they mature and develop the necessary skills and confidence. Provide age-appropriate guidance, supervision, and encouragement to help adolescents take on increasing responsibility for monitoring blood sugar, administering insulin, and making lifestyle choices.

6. School-Based Support:
   - Collaborate with school personnel to develop individualized diabetes management plans (DMPs) for children with diabetes attending school. Ensure that school staff are trained in diabetes awareness, emergency procedures, and insulin administration, and provide accommodations and support to help children participate fully in school activities while managing their diabetes safely.

7. Growth and Development Monitoring:
   - Monitor children and adolescents with diabetes for growth and developmental milestones, including height, weight, puberty, and bone health. Adjust treatment plans as needed to accommodate changes in insulin sensitivity, nutritional requirements, and physical activity levels during periods of growth and development.

8. Peer Support and Social Activities:
   - Encourage children and adolescents with diabetes to participate in peer support groups, diabetes camps, and

social activities where they can connect with others facing similar challenges and share experiences. Peer support fosters a sense of belonging, reduces feelings of isolation, and promotes adherence to diabetes self-care behaviors.

9. Long-Term Health Monitoring:
  - Provide ongoing monitoring and follow-up care to children and adolescents with diabetes to assess their long-term health outcomes, including glycemic control, cardiovascular risk factors, and diabetes-related complications. Regular screening for comorbidities and early intervention are essential for optimizing health outcomes and quality of life.

10. Transition to Adult Care:
  - Help adolescents with diabetes transition to adult diabetes care providers as they reach adulthood and prepare for independent management of their condition. Facilitate seamless transitions by providing continuity of care, preparing adolescents for adult healthcare settings, and addressing any concerns or anxieties they may have about transitioning to adult care.

By addressing these considerations and providing comprehensive, family-centered care, healthcare providers can support the health and well-being of children and adolescents with diabetes, empower them to manage their condition effectively, and promote positive outcomes for their future.

   - **Older Adults**

Older adults with diabetes require specialized care that takes into account the unique challenges associated with aging, comorbidities, cognitive changes, and functional limitations. Here are some key considerations for healthcare providers when addressing diabetes care in older adults:

1. Individualized Treatment Goals:
   - Set individualized treatment goals for older adults with diabetes, considering their overall health status, life expectancy, functional status, and personal preferences. Emphasize quality of life, functional

independence, and prevention of diabetes-related complications when establishing treatment targets.

2. Comprehensive Geriatric Assessment:
   - Conduct a comprehensive geriatric assessment to evaluate older adults with diabetes for age-related conditions, including cognitive impairment, functional limitations, falls risk, polypharmacy, malnutrition, and frailty. Use validated screening tools and assessment instruments to identify and address geriatric syndromes and multidimensional health needs.

3. Simplified Treatment Regimens:
   - Simplify diabetes treatment regimens for older adults to minimize treatment burden, medication complexity, and the risk of adverse effects. Consider using fewer medications, once-daily dosing regimens, and less intensive glycemic targets to avoid hypoglycemia and medication-related complications in this population.

4. Management of Comorbidities:
   - Address comorbidities commonly seen in older adults with diabetes, such as hypertension,

dyslipidemia, cardiovascular disease, chronic kidney disease, neuropathy, and retinopathy. Coordinate multidisciplinary care to optimize management of concurrent conditions and prevent diabetes-related complications.

5. Individualized Nutrition Counseling:
   - Provide individualized nutrition counseling for older adults with diabetes, considering their nutritional needs, dietary preferences, chewing and swallowing difficulties, and risk of malnutrition. Emphasize a balanced diet rich in fruits, vegetables, whole grains, lean proteins, and healthy fats, while minimizing added sugars, salt, and processed foods.

6. Physical Activity Recommendations:
   - Encourage regular physical activity and exercise for older adults with diabetes to improve cardiovascular health, muscle strength, balance, and mobility. Tailor exercise recommendations to the individual's functional abilities, mobility limitations, and safety considerations, incorporating low-impact activities such as walking, swimming, and tai chi.

7. Medication Safety and Adherence:
  - Ensure medication safety and adherence in older adults with diabetes by conducting regular medication reviews, simplifying medication regimens, and monitoring for adverse drug reactions and drug interactions. Educate older adults and their caregivers about proper medication use, storage, administration, and side effect management.

8. Fall Prevention Strategies:
  - Implement fall prevention strategies for older adults with diabetes to reduce the risk of falls, fractures, and mobility impairment. Assess for modifiable fall risk factors, such as impaired balance, gait disturbances, vision impairment, orthostatic hypotension, and medication side effects, and implement interventions to mitigate these risks.

9. Cognitive and Mental Health Support:
  - Address cognitive and mental health concerns in older adults with diabetes, including depression, anxiety, dementia, and cognitive impairment. Screen for

cognitive decline and provide supportive interventions, cognitive rehabilitation strategies, and referrals to mental health professionals as needed to optimize mental well-being and quality of life.

10. End-of-Life Care Planning:
   - Discuss end-of-life care preferences, advance care planning, and goals of care with older adults with diabetes and their families. Respect individual preferences for palliative care, hospice services, and advance directives, and provide compassionate, person-centered care that honors the older adult's wishes and values at the end of life.

By incorporating these considerations into diabetes care for older adults, healthcare providers can optimize treatment outcomes, improve quality of life, and promote successful aging in this population. Tailored interventions that address the unique needs and preferences of older adults with diabetes empower them to live well and maintain independence while managing their condition effectively.

- **Pregnancy and Gestational Diabetes**

Pregnancy presents unique considerations for women with diabetes, particularly gestational diabetes mellitus (GDM), which is diabetes diagnosed during pregnancy. Here are key considerations for healthcare providers when addressing diabetes care during pregnancy:

1. Preconception Counseling:
   - Provide preconception counseling to women with diabetes who are planning pregnancy to optimize glycemic control and reduce the risk of adverse pregnancy outcomes. Discuss the importance of achieving target blood sugar levels before conception and the need for close monitoring and adjustment of diabetes medications during pregnancy.

2. Screening and Diagnosis:
   - Screen pregnant women for gestational diabetes using validated screening tests, such as the glucose challenge test (GCT) or oral glucose tolerance test (OGTT), typically between 24 and 28 weeks of gestation. Diagnose GDM based on established diagnostic criteria,

such as those recommended by the American Diabetes Association (ADA) or the International Association of Diabetes and Pregnancy Study Groups (IADPSG).

3. Glycemic Control:
   - Monitor and maintain optimal blood sugar levels during pregnancy to reduce the risk of maternal and fetal complications. Emphasize the importance of self-monitoring blood glucose (SMBG), dietary modifications, physical activity, and insulin therapy as needed to achieve target glycemic targets and minimize the risk of macrosomia, birth trauma, and neonatal hypoglycemia.

4. Nutritional Counseling:
   - Provide individualized nutritional counseling to women with GDM to promote healthy eating habits, weight management, and blood sugar control during pregnancy. Emphasize a balanced diet rich in fruits, vegetables, whole grains, lean proteins, and low-fat dairy products, while limiting added sugars, refined carbohydrates, and high-glycemic index foods.

5. Physical Activity Recommendations:
   - Encourage regular physical activity and exercise during pregnancy to improve insulin sensitivity, cardiovascular health, and overall well-being. Recommend low-impact activities such as walking, swimming, prenatal yoga, and stationary cycling, and tailor exercise recommendations to the individual's fitness level, medical history, and pregnancy status.

6. Fetal Monitoring and Surveillance:
   - Perform regular fetal monitoring and surveillance for women with GDM to assess fetal growth, well-being, and development throughout pregnancy. Use techniques such as ultrasound, fetal biometry, and Doppler velocimetry to monitor fetal growth, amniotic fluid levels, and placental function, and adjust management strategies accordingly.

7. Maternal Complication Prevention:
   - Prevent maternal complications associated with GDM, such as hypertensive disorders of pregnancy (e.g., preeclampsia), preterm birth, cesarean delivery, and postpartum hemorrhage, through comprehensive

prenatal care, blood pressure monitoring, and close maternal and fetal surveillance.

8. Neonatal Care and Follow-Up:
   - Provide specialized neonatal care and follow-up for infants born to mothers with GDM to monitor for neonatal hypoglycemia, macrosomia, respiratory distress syndrome, and other complications. Implement protocols for early detection, treatment, and management of neonatal hypoglycemia, and promote breastfeeding and skin-to-skin contact to support maternal-infant bonding and glucose regulation.

9. Postpartum Care and Follow-Up:
   - Offer postpartum care and follow-up for women with GDM to assess glycemic status, screen for persistent diabetes or prediabetes, and provide counseling on lifestyle modifications, contraception, breastfeeding support, and future pregnancy planning. Emphasize the importance of long-term diabetes prevention and management strategies to reduce the risk of future complications for both mother and child.

10. Interdisciplinary Collaboration:
   - Collaborate with a multidisciplinary team of healthcare providers, including obstetricians, endocrinologists, diabetes educators, nutritionists, and perinatal specialists, to provide comprehensive, coordinated care for women with GDM. Ensure seamless communication, shared decision-making, and individualized treatment planning to optimize maternal and fetal outcomes and promote healthy pregnancies.

By addressing these considerations and providing personalized, evidence-based care, healthcare providers can support women with gestational diabetes to achieve optimal pregnancy outcomes, reduce the risk of complications, and promote the health and well-being of both mother and baby. Early detection, timely intervention, and ongoing support are key to ensuring successful management of diabetes during pregnancy and beyond.

www.ingramcontent.com/pod-product-compliance
Lightning Source LLC
Chambersburg PA
CBHW051555250726
48653CB00004BA/1170